Introduction to Biomaterials

Donglu Shi

Editor

 Tsinghua University Press 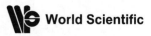 **World Scientific**

Published by

Tsinghua University Press
Xueyan Building
Tsinghua University
Beijing, 100084, P.R. China

World Scientific Publishing Co. Pte. Ltd.
5 Toh Tuck Link, Singapore 596224
USA office: 27 Warren Street, Suite 401-402, Hackensack, NJ 07601
UK office: 57 Shelton Street, Covent Garden, London WC2H 9HE

Library of Chinese Version Cataloging-in-Publications Data(2005) No. 031443
Introduction to Biomaterials   D. L. Shi
ISBN: 7-302-10807-2
Ⅰ. Bio... Ⅱ. Shi... Ⅲ Biomaterials-Colleges and Universities-Textbook-in English
Ⅳ. Q81

British Library Cataloguing-in-Publication Data
A catalogue record for this book is available from the British Library.

INTRODUCTION TO BIOMATERIALS

ISBN   7-302-10807-2/Q· 47
ISBN   981-256-627-9

Printed in China.

Introduction

In recent years, there has been increasing emphasis on materials applications in biomedical areas. However, the term "biomaterials" may have encountered different interpretations both in materials science and clinical medicine. Here we define a biomaterial as a synthetic material used to replace part of a living system or to function in intimate contact with living tissue. A biomaterial is different from a biological material, such as bone, that is produced by a biological system. Biomaterials can be categorized into different types in terms of their structural, chemical, and biological characteristics, for example, as in ceramics, glasses, and polymers with a varied degree of bioactivity. Bioma- terials represent an interdisciplinary research area that requires sufficient know- ledge of three different fields: (1) materials science and engineering processing-structure-property interrelationship of synthetic and biological materials including metals, ceramics, polymers, composites, tissues; (2) biology and physiology cell and molecular biology, anatomy, animal and human phy- siology, and (3) clinical sciences dentistry, ophthalmology, orthopedics, plastic and reconstructive surgery, cardiovascular surgery, neurosurgery, immunology, histopathology, experimental surgery, veterinary medicine and surgery.

At present, bioactive materials include some calcium phosphate compounds, bioactive glasses, bioactive glass-ceramics, bioactive ceramic coatings deposited on metal substrates, composites containing bioactive ceramic phase(s), etc. A characteristic feature common to these materials is that they bond to human bone with no fibrous tissue at the interface. Commonly, bioactivity has been defined as an ability to form an adherent interface with the tissues. The interface possesses considerable mechanical bonding and its cohesive strength is equivalent to that of the tissue and implant material. The reactions at the interface are complicated by the different responses of various types of materials.

Calcium-phosphate-based bioceramics have been in use in medicine and

I

dentistry for more than 20 years. The interest in one group member, hydroxyapatite(HA), arises from its similarity to bone apatite, the major component of the inorganic phase of bone, which plays a key role in the calcification and resorption processes of bone. The stable phases of calcium phosphate ceramics depend significantly on temperature and the presence of water, either during materials processing or in the application environment. At body temperature, only two calcium phosphates are stable when in contact with aqueous media such as body fluid(BE). The term apatite describes a family of compounds having similar structures but not necessarily having identical compositions. Biological apatites constitute the mineral phase of calcified tissues such as bone, dentin and enamel in the body and also some pathological calcifications. Biological apatites, which comprise the mineral phases of calcified tissues (enamel, dentin, bone) and of some pathological calcifications (e. g. human dental calculi, salivary stones), are usually referred to as calcium hydroxyapatite. The biological apatites are similar to synthetic hydroxyapatite (HA) but they differ from HA in composition, stoichiometry, and physical and mechanical properties. Biological apatites are usually calcium-deficient as a result of various substitutions in regular HA lattice points. HA, as noted before, is a compound of a definite composition, $Ca_{10}(PO_4)_6(OH)_2$, and a definite crystal structure. HA has been routinely used in orthopaedic surgery in both powder and bulk forms.

The current trend of developing bioactive materials has motivated an increasing need for developing biomaterials in a variety of applications. Indeed, it is clear that to achieve highly bioactive and mechanically compatible artificial materials for hard tissue prosthetics and tissue engineering(TE), it is necessary to seek for novel synthesis routes by which ideal materials can be developed with required bioactivity, porosity, microstructure, and mechanical properties. In the past, great efforts have been focused on developing metallic, ceramic, and polymer materials that could interfacially and bioactively bond to hard tissues. For instance, coating of bioactive materials onto various dense alloys and ceramics has been an effective approach in the development of bio-composite materials. However, as a result of extremely high strength and rigidity of these materials, they are not mechanically compatible with the hard tissues. On the other hand, the commonly used bioactive material HA is extremely weak in its porous form and cannot be used as structural bones. In these conventional materials, the properties cannot be easily, structurally and synthetically adjusted for bone implant. It is, therefore, highly desirable to develop a variety of bioactive materials whose structures and properties can be simulated to a real human bone.

Bioactive HA film has been coated onto porous ceramic substrates such as an industrial porous alumina (or reticulated alumina). Alumina is not only bio-inert but also mechanically strong which makes it an ideal substrate for bone substitute. The high porosity is achieved via a sponge technique by which both pore size and density can be changed easily. The bioactivity is induced by coating a HA film onto the inner pore surfaces of the reticulated alumina. Although the ceramic coating has been established on some dense substrates, it poses a great challenge in coating inner surfaces of pores as the coating area is not only partially enclosed in the material's matrix but also curved. No previous studies have so far been reported on coating inner surfaces of small-diameter pores ranging from 0.1 – 1.0 mm. The key materials processing issues dealt with in this book include precursor chemistry, coating procedures, synthesis of coated component, interface structure study, film adhesion strength testing, and mechanical properties of the component. In addition, to determine the applicability of the coated component in hard tissue prosthetics, a bioactivity study has been presented. By immersing the synthetic HA into simulated body fluid (SBF), the bioresponse has been measured for a variety of samples with different processing conditions. Significant conclusive remarks have been drawn from these extensive experiments that this novel approach has shown great promise in synthesizing structural artificial bones for hard tissue prosthe-tics. The fabricated components can be designed and synthesized to have similar properties comparable to human bones in terms of porosity, mechanical strength, and bioactivity. Furthermore, fundamental aspects of this research are centered on the effects of structural characteristics of HA on bioactivity. Based on extensive infrared spectroscopy (IR) and X-ray diffraction (XRD) experimental data, it has been found that the bioactivity of HA is sensitively controlled by the structural crystallinity of the HA and its specific surface area. A physical model has been developed to interpret the observed phenomena.

Polymers have been widely used as biomaterials for the fabrication of medical device and tissue engineering scaffolds. Naturally occurring polymers, synthetic non-biodegradable and synthetic biodegradable polymers are the main types of polymers used as biomaterials. Naturally occurring polymers, such as collagen, chitin and starch, are an important class of biomaterials due to their biodegradation characteristics and plentiful availability. Synthetic polymers represent the majority of the polymer biomaterials — from traditional engineering plastics to newly engineered biomaterials for specific biomedical applications. Although most synthetic non-biodegradable polymers were originally designed for non-biomedical use, they are widely used as biomaterials mainly because of their desirable physical-mechanical properties. There are still no newly engineered biomaterials, which can replace these "old" polymers. A good example is Polymethyl metacrylate (PMMA) bone cement, which has been used since

1943 and is still being widely used clinically nowadays. Synthetic biodegradable polymers have attracted much attention in the last decade because the biodegradable polymers can be eliminated from the human body after fulfilling their intended purpose and therefore a second surgery can be avoided. Also, the emergence of tissue engineering has demanded the use of biodegradable scaffolds for the regeneration of tissues and organs. A lot of biodegradable polymers are derived from the traditional polymers by introducing non-stable chemical linkages, such as hydrolysable ester bonds.

The use of biomaterials in orthopedic surgeries represents a significant challenge to biomaterials scientists. Biomaterials for orthopedic use will have to possess sufficient mechanical properties for sharing or bearing the load. They will also need to be able to bond to host bone (bone-bonding). Ideally, the biomaterials will be gradually replaced by newly formed bone during the wound healing process. One of the solutions is to use bioactive ceramics, such as calcium phosphate and Bioglass^{TM}, to reinforce polymers so that the mechanical properties and the bone-bonding properties of the polymer can be improved.

This book gives a comprehensive introduction to most of the important biomaterials including ceramics, metals, and polymers from a fundamental point of view, which is suitable for both undergraduate and graduate students. Part I mainly deals with critical issues in bioceramics and metals in the areas of synthesis methods, characterization techniques, mechanical property analysis, heat treatment, and *in vitro* bioactivity test. Most recent experimental results on the coating of HA onto porous ceramics and their bioactivity study are included in Chapter 2 through Chapter 7. These chapters should interest many researchers in this field. An introduction to metallic biomaterials is included in Chapter 8. Part II addresses the important problems in polymers and their applications in medical fields. Part II is entirely dedicated to tissue engineering, which is closely related to Parts I and II. Not only are these chapters well referenced with the most up-to-date publications, but also followed with exercise problems and questions for classroom lecturing.

Biomaterials research has been advancing rapidly in recent years, particularly in the field of tissue engineering. The research addresses the critical issues in medical applications including bioactivity, compatibility, toxicity, and mechanical properties of all types of biomaterials. In the biomedical applications, traditional materials science and engineering have to deal with new challenges in the areas of synthesis, microstructure development, and biological, chemical, and physical behaviors, since medical needs place new demands in these respects.

The most fascinating development in biomaterials is to be found in tissue engineering, and involves the direct use of material within a biological system.

Today, tissue-engineered skin is already available on the market; and tissue-engineered cartilage is undergoing clinical trials and should be available within a few years. Temporary liver-assistance devices are also being clinically tested. Tissue-engineered bone is not very far behind. Up to now, investigators have attempted to build bone, liver, arteries, bladder, pancreas, nerves, cartilage, heart valves, cornea, and various soft tissues. Despite significant progress in this field, a number of issues have arisen that force the commercial process to take a breather. By simply producing highly porous scaffold and seeding it with appropriate cell types, one cannot in most cases obtain the desired features of a normal tissue. The challenge for future tissue engineering concerns how subcellular structures dictate cell function. We need to know how to fabricate organ-scale structures with cellular resolution, integrating functional cells to yield a 3-D architecture for tissue function. This is necessary to integrate the tissue into patients with the desired vascularization and controlled immune responses.

A typical tissue engineering device comprises cells and scaffolds. Typically, in the construction, biological materials (cells and cellular products) provide the biological function whereas synthetic materials give the structural support. Ideally, the interaction results in the integration of the device with the host, maintenance of the biological function, and control of signals between device and host. Biomaterials have been used as supporting scaffold for the growth of cellular components. The materials can vary from polymers to bioceramics. One interesting trend in developing biomaterials for scaffolds is to design specialized biomaterials. For example, one can design a material that erodes to naturally occurring byproducts *in vivo* (temporary scaffold), incorporate bioactive moieties to facilitate tissue in-growth and host response, block undesirable biological phenomena, and alter material properties in response to environmental stimuli (smart materials). The scaffold should provide the physicochemical signals to control cellular interactions, give structural support, and also provide sites for cell attachment, migration, and tissue in-growth. Biomaterial microstructure is often dictated by process parameters such as the choice of solvent in phase separation, doping with leachants, controlled ice crystal formation and subsequent freeze-drying to create pores. Almost all these techniques are very sensitive to processing parameters. The other important issue in biomaterials is the scaffold chemistry patterning. Scaffold may incorporate specific bioactive chemical moieties to direct cell adhesion, migration, and tissue in-growth and repair. A precisely defined scaffold depends on the development of a novel biomaterial tailored to specific physicochemical material properties and structures.

Despite extensive research activities in biomaterials and tissue engineering, there have been a few comprehensive textbooks that systematically introduce the fundamental concepts in all types of materials including metallic, ceramic, and polymer materials in terms of their synthesis, structure, and bioactive behaviors. Further, closely related materials applications in tissue engineering are not entirely combined with the introduction of specific biomaterials in a textbook.

University students and researchers can benefit from this book in diversified backgrounds such as orthopedics, biochemistry, biomedical engineering, materials science, tissue engineering, and other related medical fields. Both undergraduate and graduate students will find the book a valuable reference not only on biomaterial, but also on tissue engineering-related topics, including biostructures and phase diagrams of complex systems, hard tissue prosthetics, novel biomaterials processing methods, and new materials-characterization techniques. Thus, it can serve as a comprehensive introduction to researchers in biomaterials science and engineering in general, and can also be used as a graduate-level text in related areas.

This book is written by several prominent scholars in the fields of biomaterials and TE. Chapters 1 – 7 are mainly written by Dr. Donglu Shi on bioceramics based on his lecture notes from a biomaterials class that he has taught at the University of Cincinnati. Some of the recent experimental research results are obtained from his laboratory at the University of Cincinnati. His formal PhD student, Dr. Gengwei Jiang was intensely involved in these experiments and mainly responsible for the data presented in these chapters. Donglu Shi is most grateful to her dedicated work and appreciates the extensive previous results used in Chapters 1 – 7. Dr. Xuejun Wen has not only written the chapters with Dr. Ning Zhang in Part III on tissue engineering, but also co-authored with Donglu Shi in writing Chapter 2 and Chapter 3 on the fundamentals of bioceramics. Dr. Yang Leng is a well known scholar in biomaterials and responsible for Chapter 8 on metallic materials. Finally, Dr. Qing Liu has authored Part II on bio-polymers. In Chapter 1, part of the definitions of biomaterials is from a book chapter by Prof. M. Wang ("Biomaterials and Tissue Engineering" ed. D. Shi, Springer-TUP, 2004). We hope these chapters will provide timely and useful information for the progress of biomaterials and clinical applications.

Contents

Part I Bioactive Ceramics and Metals

Part Ⅱ Polymeric Biomaterials

X

Part Ⅲ Tissue Engineering: A New Era of Regenerative Medicine

Part Ⅰ

Bioactive Ceramics and Metals

1 Introduction to Bioceramics[*]

1.1 Bioactive Materials

1.1.1 Definitions

In recent years, there has been increasing emphasis of materials applications in biomedical areas. However the definition of "biomaterials" may have encountered different interpretations both in materials science and clinical medicine. Biomaterial is defined as a synthetic material, which is implanted to substitute living tissue for satisfying normal functionalities of the body. Such a synthetic material with certain bioactivity, from a biological point of view, is fundamentally different from a biological soft or hard tissue such as bone, dentin, and enamel in the body.

As a characteristic of 21st century science, research on biomaterials intensely involves interdisciplinary collaboration from several major areas and requires extensive knowledge in medical science, materials science, biochemistry, biomedical engineering and clinical science. As biomaterials mainly deal with all aspect materials synthesis and processing, knowledge in materials science and engineering is essential. Therefore all fundamentals in materials synthesis, processing, structure, and properties are needed in carrying out research in biomaterials. However, biomaterials research places great emphasis on biological responses and biochemistry reactions of the synthesized materials, the study on property-structure relationship, a common topic in engineering materials, may focus more on biological behaviors, rather then engineering properties. On the other hand, as the main purposes of the biomaterials are in clinical applications, biomedical sciences become an important part of research in biomaterials. These include cell and molecular biology, anatomy, and animal and human physiology. For instance, during implant, the interface between substitute biomaterial and biological tissue is the central issue, which must be studied

---

* Authors are Donglu Shi and Gengwei Jiang.

from point views of both materials and biological/physiological sciences. Biomaterials have been widely used in many clinical applications such as orthopedics, dentistry, plastic and reconstructive surgery, ophthalmology, cardiovascular surgery, neurosurgery, immunology, histopathology, experimental surgery, and veterinary medicine and surgery. Therefore, knowledge and expertise in these areas become essential in biomaterials research.

Hench and Ethridge have defined biomaterials as: "a bioactive material is one that elicits a specific biological response at the interface of the material which results in the formation of a bond between the tissues and the material" [1]. Studies have shown that the materials that exhibit bioactivity include some calcium phosphate compounds, bioactive glasses, bioactive glass-ceramics, and composites with these materials. A common feature shared by these materials is that they all, to certain degree, bond to human bone by forming an interface between the implant and the tissue.

1.1.2　Common Biomaterials

In this book, the "biomaterials" is the "bioactive material", which excludes an others nonbioactive engineering structured materials. Bioactivity has been defined as an ability to form an adherent interface with the tissues. The interface between the hard tissue and the implant materials possesses considerable mechanical bonding and cohesive strength. The reactions at the interface exhibit different responses from various types of materials. The common bioactive materials can be classified by their bioreactivities and reaction mechanisms. According to Hench $(2 - 7)$, the following materials all exhibit bioreactivity, however, with a varied degree: 45S5, KGS Ceravital, 55S4.3 Bioglass, A-W GC, HA, KGX Ceravital. 45S5 and 55S4.3 were name by Hench, which contain SiO_2, CaO, Na_2O, and P_2O_2 in certain specific proportions. KGS and KGX are glass-ceramics containing apatite, named by Gross [8]. A-W GC stands for apatite- and wollastonite (CaO SiO)-containing glass-ceramics. Al_2O_3 and Si_3N_4, although nearly bio-inner, are also used as implant materials. The reaction of these bioactive materials takes place only at surfaces and the boning has been known to be a chemical process. As a result of relatively low bioreactivities of hydroxyapatite (HA) and KGX Ceravital, their boning to bone is through porous intergrowth. Al_2O_3 and Si_3N_4 have been found to be biocompatible with the tissues. On the other hand, tricalcium phosphate (TCP) is classified as bioresorable. Ceramics of this type exhibits high bioreactivity and can make a direct contact with bone forming a mechanical bonding.

1.1.3　Bioactive Ceramics

Calcium phosphate-based bioceramics have been used in clinical applications for more than 20 years. Due to the similarity between hydroxyapatite and bone apatite, it has played a key role in the calcification and resorption processes of bone [9]. Jarcho *et al.* in the USA, de Groot *et al.* in Europe, and Aoki *et al.* in Japan worked in 1970's towards the development and commercialization of hydroxyapatite as a biomaterial for bone repair, augmentation and substitution.

The phase stabilities of calcium phosphate ceramics have been found to be associated with processing temperature, the presence of water, and biological environment. Only two calcium phosphates are stable when in contact with aqueous media such as body fluids at body temperature. The stable phase is $CaHPO_4 \cdot 2H_2O$ (brushite) at pH < 4.2, while the stable phase is $Ca_{10}(PO_4)_6(OH)_2(HA)$ at pH >4.2. Other phases such as $Ca_3(PO_4)_2(TCP)$ and $Ca_4P_2O_9(TTCP)$ may appear at higher temperatures. When in contact with water or body fluids at $37°C$, the unhydrated high-temperature calcium phosphate phases may react to form HA.

It has been observed that the β-TCP: HA ratio plays a key role in biphasic calcium phosphate materials; the higher the ratio, the greater the abundance of the CO_3^{-} apatite micro-crystals, which are contained on the surfaces of the large BCP crystals. This has been found to be associated with the higher dissolution properties of the β-TCP component of the BCP. The high dissolution rate leads to an increase in the concentration of the calcium and phosphate ions in the microenvironment, which causes precipitation of the carbonated apatite.

1.1.4　Biological Apatites

The term apatite implies a group of compounds having similar structures but not necessarily having identical compositions. Bone, dentin and enamel in the body all contain biological apatites, which comprise the mineral phases of calcified tissues. They are normally referred to as calcium hydroxyapatite. Although the biological apatites are similar to synthetic hydroxyapatite (HA), they present differences in composition, stoichiometry, and physical and mechanical properties. Biological apatites are usually calcium-deficient due to various substitutions in regular HA lattice points. Therefore both biological apatite and synthetic hydroxyapatite should not be confused and interchangeably used as their definitions are significantly different. HA, as noted before, is a compound of a specific composition, $Ca_{10}(PO_4)_6(OH)_2$, with a well defined crystal structure.

1.1.5 Basic Requirements for Bone Implants

A bioactive material is defined as a material that induces a specific biological response at the interface of the material that results in the formation of a bond between the tissues and the implant materials. As identified previously, many ceramics and glasses are bioactive. In particular, in the calcium phosphate system, hydroxyapatite (HA) ($Ca_{10}(PO_4)_6(OH)_2$) exhibit good biological stability and affinity. A common characteristic of all bioactive implants is the formation of a hydroxy-carbonate apatite (HCA) layer on their surface when implanted. The HCA phase is equivalent in composition and structure to the mineral phase of bone. The HCA layer grows as polycrystalline. Collagen fibrils are incorporated within the agglomerates thereby binding the inorganic implant surface to the organic constituents of tissues.

As a result of its good tissue response, HA has been routinely used in orthopaedic surgery in both powder and bulk forms. However, their weak mechanical properties preclude their use in load-bearing situations. The best solution to this problem is using HA as a coating on alloys or high strength ceramics, combining the strength of a substrate with the osteoconductive capacity of HA. Industrial and laboratory techniques used for coating HA onto dense metallic and ceramic substrates include plasma spraying, electrophotetic deposition, sputtering and hot isostatic pressing (10 – 12). In all previous work, however, coating of HA on a mechanically strong substrate has been limited to dense bulk materials, such as metallic alloys and ceramics. The critical problems associated with a dense material in hard tissue prosthetics are significantly reduced surface areas and low porosity that are essential in bone growth.

In the development of bone substitutes, high porosity level is required for the following considerations:

(1) Porous materials have large surface area, resulting in a high tendency to bioresorb, which induces high bioactivity.

(2) Interconnected pores permit tissue ingrowth and thus anchor the prosthesis with the surrounding bone, preventing loosening of implants.

Interconnected porosity acts like an organization of vascular canals which can ensure the blood and nutrition supply for the bone. For serving this purpose, it is required that the dimension of the interconnected system is at least 100 μm in diameter. According to these requirements, reticulated alumina has been chosen as the substrate material. Note that many other types of reticulated cer-amics can also be used as substrate including ZrO_2 and MgO since they are chemically stable and mechanically strong. The most common applications of porous ceramics, also called reticulated ceramics, are molten-metal and diesel engine exhaust filters [13]. It can also be used as catalyst supports and industrial hot-gas filters, thermal insulators, and gas combustion burners. Structurally, a reticulated material is a porous matrix comprising interconnected voids surrounded by a web of ceramic, metal, or polymer as shown in Fig. 1.1. These porous network structures have relatively low mass, low density, and low thermal conductivity. The open-cell nature of reticulated materials is a unique characteristic essential in many applications. However, the surface-to-volume ratio of reticulated materials is much larger that of the dense materials, making them ideal for surface reaction applications.

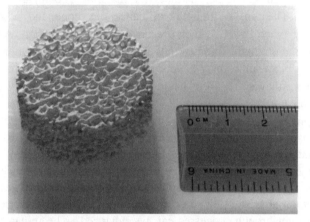

Figure 1.1 Reticulated alumina with a high level of porosity

The control of porosity is obtained by the polymeric-sponge method [13]. The method was originally developed for making reticulated ceramics with a porous structure comprising interconnected voids surrounded by a web of ceramic. The processing route involves the following steps: (1) Selection of sponge. Certain sponge materials are selected for processing reticulated ceramics including poly(urethane), cellulose, poly(vinyl chloride, poly(styrene), and latex; (2) Preparation of slurry containing substrate ceramics. The slurry is made of ceramic powders, water, and additives which are commercially available; (3) Immerse of slurry in sponge. The sponge is immersed in slurry and allowed to expand; (4) Drying. The sponge filled with slurry is dried in air in a temperature range between 100°C and 700°C; (5) Burn out of polymeric sponge. The dried sponge is heated to between 350°C and 800°C to burn out the organics from the slurry, and (6) Sintering.

A typical reticulated ceramic (alumina) is shown in Fig. 1.1. Using the sponge method many reticulated materials can now be readily processed into a variety of geometry. These include Al_2O_3, Fe_3O_4, ZrO_2, and SiC. Their strength can also be modified by altering the pore density, size, and distribution.

1.1.6 Coating of Hydroxyapatite on Porous Ceramics

The weak mechanical properties of bioceramics such as HA have been the primary obstacles to the applications in hard tissue prosthetics. It has been reported that the strength of the porous bioactive materials is comparable to the cancellous bone. The tensile strengths of cancellous bone and porous calcium phosphates are much lower, which are on the order of 5 MPa. As a result of poor mechanical strength, biomaterials are precluded from common structural bones. Dense bioceramics may have significantly improved mechanical properties. However, they suffer from having much lower bioreactivity due to smaller surface area.

To improve the mechanical strength, various methods have been developed such as glass-ceramics composite [14, 15]. However, all these strengthened materials are dense with low, or zero porosity, which may not be desirable in many prosthetic applications. Low porosity will lead to much slower dissolution rates, and in turn adversely affect the bioresorbability and reactivity. Only when a large amount of pores are introduced into the materials, reaction kinetics and inter-growth processes can be enhanced. The research work conducted specifically deals with these important issues by a novel approach. To enhance the mechanical properties, an industrial alumina has been selected as the substrate. Alumina is not only bio-inert but also mechanically strong which makes it an ideal substrate for bone substitute. The high porosity is achieved via a sponge technique by which both pore size and density can be changed easily. The bioactivity is induced coating a HA film onto the inner pore surfaces of reticulated alumina. This new approach is a major topic in the research work presented.

The basic idea of the novel approach is illustrated in Fig. 1.2. To satisfy the basic requirements in bone implant, we need: (1) a high porosity level for an organization of vascular canals that can ensure the blood supply; (2) compatible mechanical properties with bone structure, and (3) a high bioactivity for bone ingrowth. The substrate of the composite is a strong, bio-inert porous matrix, which provides the mechanical strength needed for the structural bone. The strength can also be altered by changing the dimension and density of the porosity, so that the composite is mechanically compatible to the human bone. A highly bioactive material, namely, hydroxyapatite (HA) is coated onto the inner surfaces of the pores in the substrate. In this way, the hard tissue can be in contact with a large surface area that is bioactive. Bone ingrowth is well induced due to the high porosity level and coated bioactive surface areas. Figure 1.2 schematically illustrate the HA-coated pore surfaces.

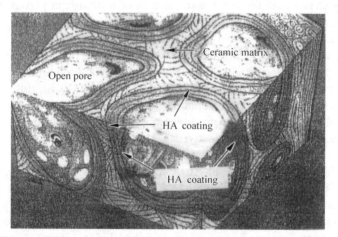

Figure 1.2 The porous matrix with inner pore surfaces coated with HA

Although the ceramic coating has been established on some dense substrates, it poses a great challenge in coating inner surfaces of pores as the coating area is not only partially enclosed in the material's matrix but also curved. No previous studies have so far been reported on coating inner surfaces of small-diameter pores ranging from 0.1 – 1.0 mm. The key materials processing issues dealt with precursor chemistry, coating procedures, synthesis of coated component, interface structure study, film adhesion strength testing, and mechanical properties of the component. In addition, to determine the applicability of the coated component in hard tissue prosthetics, a bioactivity study has been carried out. By immersing the synthetic HA into simulated body fluid (SBF), the bioresponse has been measured for a variety of samples with different processing conditions. Significant conclusive remarks have been drawn from these extensive experiments that this novel approach has shown great promise in synthesizing structural artificial bones for hard tissue prosthetics. The fabricated components can be designed and synthesized to have similar properties comparable to human bones in terms of porosity, mechanical strength, and bioactivity. Furthermore, fundamental aspects of this research are centered on the effects of structural characteristics of HA on the bioactivity.

Based on extensive infra-red (IR) and X-ray diffraction (XRD) experimental data, it has been found that the bioactivity of HA is sensitively controlled by the structural crystallinity of the HA and its specific surface area. A physical model has been developed to interpret the observed phenomena.

The purpose of current research is several-fold. Firstly, the aim is to develop an effective method by which a bioactive material, namely, HA, will be uniformly coated onto the inner pore surfaces of a strong but porous matrix. In this current work reticulated alumina has been chosen as shown in Fig. 1. 3, which is an industrially viable and mechanically strong ceramic. Three major coating techniques have been developed for this purpose — sol-gel, suspension, and thermal deposition, and all of which will be introduced later in detail. All these methods have proved effective, however, with different procedures depending upon specific applications. Secondly, interface structures and mechanical properties have been studied that are important in developing other types of porous and bioactive materials. This has allowed an understanding on the new mechanisms in coating an inner surface with a varied curvature. Thirdly, a detailed understanding of physical mechanisms underlying bioactivity of the HA composites has been established. The composite HA with a large pore density, considering its high surface energies, is expected to have greatly enhanced bioactivity compared to its conventional counterparts. However, such a new reaction mechanism has never been studied before. The HA-coated composite can possess a wide range of pore density, therefore exhibiting new bioactivity behaviors, which can be fine-tuned by the pore structure. The bioactivity study has shown that the bioactivity of HA is strongly affected by its structural characteristics and specific surface area.

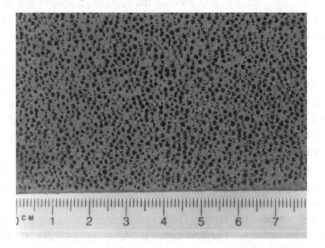

Figure 1. 3 A reticulated alumina as the substrate with a high porosity level

1.1.7 Biomaterials in Tissue Attachment

Previous studies have shown that the bone mineral crystals are not pure hydroxyapatite (HA) ($Ca_{10}(PO_4)_6(OH_2)_2$), but acid phosphate groups (HPO_4^{2-}) and carbonate ions. Therefore, they may be best classified as appatite rather than HA. Mineralization of bone is an important process in bone activities. It involves a sequence of changes in composition and density in an organized fashion. During such a process, the solid calcium phosphate is formed with an increased stiffness in bone structure. Although it plays an important role in bone biology, the chemical and biological mechanisms during mineralization have not been well understood.

The attachment of tissues to an implant is directly related to the tissue response at the implant interface. There are four types of bioceramics, each with a different type of tissue attachment:

Type 1 — Nearly inert, implant does not form a bond with bone. Instead, the fibrous tissue is formed in order to "wall off" or isolate the implant from the host. It is a protective mechanism and with time can lead to complete encapsulation of an implant within the fibrous layer. Alumina, zirconia, metals and most polymers produce this type of interfacial response.

Type 2 — Porous, implant forms a mechanical bond via ingrowth of bone into the pores. The growth of bone into surface porosity provides a large interfacial area between the implant and its host, preventing loosening of implants. It is capable of withstanding more complex stress states than type 1 implants. A typical example of porous implant is porous hydroxyapatite (HA).

Type 3 — Bioactive, implant forms a bond with bone via chemical reactions at the interface. A common characteristic of all bioactive implants is the formation of a hydroxy-carbonate apatite (HCA) layer on their surface when implanted. The thickness of reaction layer among different materials ranges from 0.5 – 100 μm, which is likely due to the difference in their solubility. Examples of bioactive implants include HA and bioactive glasses.

Type 4 — Resorbable, implant degrades gradually with time and is replaced by bone. A very thin or non-existent interfacial thickness is the final result. For a successful application of this kind of materials, the resorption rates must match the repair rates of body tissues, and the mechanical performance should also be compatible while regeneration of tissues is occurring. Examples of resorbable implants include tricalcium phosphate, bioactive glasses and specially formulated polymers.

1.2 References

1. Hench, L. L. , E. C. Ethridge. Biomaterials: An Interfacial Approach. Academic Press, New York (1982)
2. Hench, L. L. J. Non-Crystalline Solids. **19**: 27 (1975)
3. Hench, L. L. Stability of ceramics in the physiological eniroment. In: D. F. Williams, ed. Fundamental Aspects of Biocompatibility. Vol. 1. FL CRC Press, Boca Raton, p. 67 (1981)
4. Hench, L. L. J. de Physique. **43**: C9 (1982)
5. Hench, L. L. Bioactive ceramics. Ann. N. Y. Acad. Sci. **523**: 54 (1988)
6. Hench, L. L. J. Non-Crystalline Solids. **28**: 79 (1978)
7. Hench, L. L., A. E. Clark. Adhesion to Bone, Biocompatibility of Orthopaedic Implants. Vol. 2. CRC Press, Boca Raton, p. 129 (1982)
8. Van Raemdonk, W., P. J. Ducheyne. Am Ceram. Soc. **6**: 381 (1984)
9. Fawcett, D. W. A Textbook of Histology. W. B. Company, London (1986)
10. de Groot, K. Hydroxyapatite coating for implant in surgery. In: P. Vincezini, ed. High Tech Ceramics. Elsevier, Amsterdam, pp. 381 – 390 (1987)
11. Van Raemdonck, W., P. Ducheyne. Auger electron spectroscopic analysis of hydroxyapatite coatings on titanium. J. Am. Ceram. Soc. **6**(2): 381 – 384 (1984)
12. Pilliar, R., H. Cameron. Porous surface layered prosthetic devices. BioMed. Eng. **10** (10): 126 – 135 (1975)
13. Saggio-Woyansky, J., C. E. Scott, W. P. Minnear. American Ceramic Society Bulletin. **71**: 1674 (1992)
14. Santos, J. D. , J. C. Knowles, S. Morrey, F. J. Monterio, G. W. Hastings. Biocertamics, **5**: 35 – 41 (1992)
15. Knowles, J. C. , W. Bonfield. J. Biomed. Mater. Res. **27**: 1591 – 1598 (1993)

2 Bioactive Ceramics: Structure, Synthesis, and Mechanical Properties[*]

In order to substitute the function of lost or damaged hard tissues, such as bone and tooth, tissue transplants and synthetic devices have been utilized. Tissue transplants can be autologous, allogeneic, or xenogeneic. However, the use of autologous tissue involves additional surgery and donor site morbidity; and the use of allogeneic or xenogeneic tissue involves the risks of immune rejection and disease transmission [1, 2]. Therefore, synthetic hard tissue implants are very necessary. All categories of biomaterials including metals, ceramics, composites, and even polymers are investigated as candidates for the hard tissue replacements. For heavy loaded applications, such as hip prostheses, metals (e.g. Ti-alloys, Co—Cr, etc.) and strong inert ceramics (e.g. alumina, zirconia, etc.) are extensively studied [1, 2]. Unfortunately, various problems related to both the metallic materials and the bio-inert ceramics are evident, for example, corrosion, elastic modulus mismatch (stress concentration and shielding), and bioinertness (only physical connection with host) with metals, and brittle, elastic modulus mismatch, and bioinertness with bio-inert ceramics [3]. For these reasons, bioactive ceramics, mainly including calcium phosphates and bioactive glasses, are showing very promising results in the high bioactivity and the formation of interfacial chemical bond with host tissue, which was called osseointegration. The advantages of bioactive ceramics over inert ceramics and metals allow for developing second generation of hard tissue substitutions with the characteristics of bioactive and equal elastic modulus when compared with bone. On the other hand, the mechanical properties of bioceramics are fairly poor when compared with their replaced natural hard tissues. The poor mechanical properties, especially inside the body aqueous environments, highly limit their applications to only small, unloaded, and low-loaded implants, powders, coatings, composites, porous scaffolds for tissue engineering, and so on. Interestingly, bioactive ceramic coatings and porous scaffold are showing the most promising results for the future hard tissue replacements

---

[*] Authors are Donglu Shi and Xuejun Wen.

[4 – 6], which can be named as the third generation of hard substitutes. So far, several bioactive ceramics have been proposed for hard tissue replacements, from the biocompatibility point of view, hydroxyapatide (HA) and bioactive glasses are the most acceptable materials for hard tissue applications [3, 4, 6].

2.1　Structure of Hydroxyapatite

2.1.1　General Structure and Chemistry of Hydroxyapatite

One of the most extensively studied bioactive ceramics is hydroxyapatite. Hydroxyapatite(HA) is chemically similar to the mineral component of bone and other hard tissue in mammals, i.e. it is composed of the same ions that construct the mineral part of teeth and bones. It shows excellent biocompatibility not only with hard tissues, but also with soft tissues, such as skin and muscle. Moreover, it is bioactive, and promotes osseointegration when directly implanted into bone. Before we approach the chemical structures of HA, it is of great importance to know the chemical compositions of hard tissues. For the natural bone tissue, the main components are calcium phosphate (69 wt%), water (10 wt%), collagen (20 wt%) and other organic materials in small quantities, such as proteins, polysaccharides, and lipids as shown in Fig. 2.1. Collagen is in the shape of tiny filaments with its diameter ranging from 0.1 μm to 2 μm. The main function of collagen is elasticity and structure support to the bone tissue. Calcium phosphate is in the form of crystallized HA and amorphous calcium phosphate (ACP). The main function is providing stiffness to the bone tissue. The HA crystals, in the form of needles and plates, are parallel to the collagen filaments [7]. In the natural teeth, there are three different types of hard tissue: enamel, dentine, and cementum. The enamel is the hardest substance in the body and consists of 97 wt% crystal HA and 3 wt% organic substance and water. The dentine has the composition very similar to bone tissue. The cementum is composed of 45 wt% minerals and 55 wt% organic materials and water [8]. In human body, the most important calcium phosphates are HA with a Ca:P ratio of 1.67 and tricalcium phosphate (TCP) with a Ca:P ratio of 1.5 [7].

　　Pure stoichiometric HA ($Ca_{10}(PO_4)_6(OH)_2$) consists of Ca^{2+}, PO_4^{2-}, and OH^- ions. The lattice structure of apatite is schematically shown in Fig. 2.2. Ca^{2+} form column structures and OH^- ions reside inside the channels.

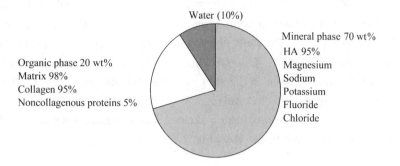

Figure 2.1 Composition of bone

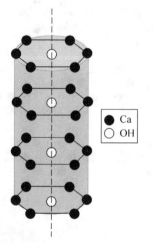

Figure 2.2 The simplified lattice structure of apatite

2.1.2   Structural Characteristics of Hydroxyapatite

The structure of HA belongs to the hexagonal system with a $P6_3/m$ space group. The overall arrangement of HA is characterized by a c-axis perpendicular to 3 equivalent a-axis at angle $120°$ to each other. The unit cell, the smallest building unit and a complete representation of the HA crystal, consists of Ca^{2+}, PO_4^{2-} and OH^- groups closely packed together in a hexagonal arrangement as shown in Fig. 2.3. According to the position in the unit cell, ten calcium (Ca) atoms can be classified into two types: Ca_1 and Ca_2. Four calcium atoms occupy the Ca_1 positions, which locate in an octahedral site of a hexagonal array, and six calcium atoms live in Ca_2 position, which locates at the corners of the hexagonal column and surrounds the OH^- ions. However, six Ca_2 atoms are not in the same plane, each three arrange in triangle positions at $z = 0.25$ and at $z = 0.75$. The OH^- ions are located in the centerline of the hexagonal channel. Similar to the six Ca_2 atoms, the six phosphates (PO_4) are in a helical arrangement from levels $z = 0.25$ to $z = 0.75$ and arrange in two triangles as well. PO_4 groups form a skeletal frame structural network, which provides structural stability for HA (Fig. 2.3) [1, 3, 7].

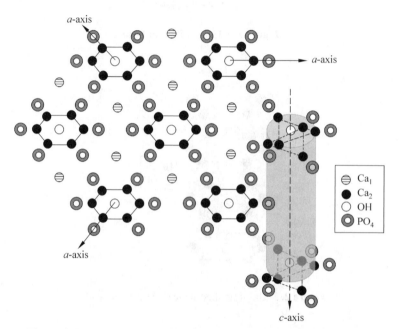

Figure 2.3 The atomic arrangement of calcium HA, $Ca_{10}(PO_4)_6(OH)_2$

2.1.3   Substituted Apatite

However, the biological hydroxyapatite (HA) in the body differs from that of pure HA in stoichiometry, composition, physical properties and mechanical properties, became this HA is particularly prone to ion substitution. The biological HA is usually calcium-deficient (i.e. the Ca : P molar ratio is lower than the stoichiometric value of 1.67 for pure HA) and is always carbonate substituted. Substitutions may involve ions of Mg^{2+}, Na^+, K^+, Sr^{2+}, or Ba^{2+} for

Ca^{2+}, CO_3^{2-}, $H_2PO_4^-$, HPO_4^{2-}, and SO_4^{2-} for PO_4^{3-}, and F^-, Cl^-, and CO_3^{2-} for OH^-. Therefore, the appropriate formula of biological HA is:

$$(Ca, \ M)_{10}(PO_4, \ Y)_6(OH, \ X)_2.$$

Where M represents other cations (e.g. Mg^{2+}, Na^+, K^+, Sr^{2+}, Ba^{2+}, etc.); Y represents carbonates, acid phosphate, HPO_4^{2-}, sulfates, etc.; while X represents F^-, Cl^-, carbonates, etc.

For example, when fluoride (F) substitutes for the OH groups in the apatite structure, F-apatite ($Ca_{10}(PO_4)_6F_2$) forms. Similarly, when chloride (Cl) substitutes for the OH groups, Cl-apatite ($Ca_{10}(PO_4)_6Cl_2$) forms. However, the positions of OH, Cl, or F in the Ca_{10} (PO_4)$_6$ $(OH)_2$ (OH-apatite), $Ca_{10}(PO_4)_6F_2$ (F-apatite) and $Ca_{10}(PO_4)_6Cl_2$ (Cl-apatite), respectively, are different as shown in Fig. 2.4, although OH, F, and Cl atoms lie along the c-axis at the center of the Ca_2 triangles.

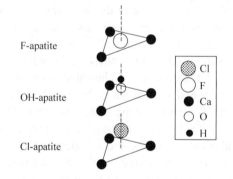

Figure 2.4 The relative positions of F, OH, and Cl atoms at the center of the Ca_2 triangles in F-apatite ($Ca_{10}(PO_4)_6F_2$), OH-apatite ($Ca_{10}(PO_4)_6(OH)_2$), and Cl-apatite ($Ca_{10}(PO_4)_6Cl_2$)

Substitution of any group in the hydroxyapatite may cause changes in characteristics, such as lattice parameters (The lattice parameters of several apatites are shown in Table 2.1), crystallinity, crystal symmetry, thermal stability, morphology, solubility, and physical, chemical and biological properties [9, 10].

2.1 Structure of Hydroxyapatite

Table 2.1 Lattice parameters of different apatites

	a-Axis	c-Axis
Human enamel HA	9.441	6.882
Synthetic HA (non-aqueous)	9.441	6.882
Synthetic HA (aqueous)	9.438	6.882
F-apatite (non-aqueous)	9.375	6.880
F-apatite (aqueous)	9.382	6.880
Cl-apatite (non-aqueous)	9.646	6.771
Cl, OH-apatite (aqueous)	9.515	6.858
CO_3 apatite (non-aqueous)	9.544	6.859
CO_3, OH-apatite (aqueous)	9.298	6.924

Fluorine (F^-) substitution for the OH^- group — The substitution of F^- for OH^- group can greatly improves the physical, chemical and biological properties of HA, such as increment in the crystallinity, decrement in the a-axis dimension without varying the c-axis, increment in crystal size and therefore lessening crystal strain, enhancement in the structural stability, improvement in corrosion resistance in biological environments, and so on. F-substituted apatites are less soluble than F-free apatites. That is why fluorine is often used in teeth paste to prevent tooth decay by increasing the stability of apatites.

Carbonate (CO_3^{2-}) substitution — The substitution of carbonate can cause a decrease in crystallinity and an increase in the extent of dissolution of apatites. Carbonate can substitute two sites: One is the hydroxyl (OH^-) site, which is designated as Type A substitution. The other is phosphate (PO_4^{3-}) site, which is called Type B substitution. Carbonate substituted HA can be fabricated as well. For example, Type A apatite could be obtained by treating pure hydroxyapatite in a dry CO_2 environment, while Type B apatite could be achieved by precipitation from aqueous solutions. In general, biological apatite is referred to as Type B. These two types of substitution have opposite effects on the lattice parameters: a-axis and c-axis dimensions. For Type A substitution, a smaller OH^- is replaced by a larger CO_3^{2-}, resulting in an expansion in the a-axis and contraction in the c-axis. For Type B substitution, a larger PO_4^{3-} is traded by a smaller CO_3^{2-}, leading to a contraction in the a-axis and expansion in the c-axis as shown in Fig. 2.5.

Substitution with other ions — Some ions, such as Mg^{2+}, Na^+, K^+, Sr^{2+}, Ba^{2+}, Pb^{2+}, etc., can replace Ca^{2+}. Other ions, such as V^{5+}, Mn^{5+}, BO_3^{3-}, etc. can substitute PO_4^{3-}. For example, Mg^{2+} causes a decrease in crystallinity and an increase in the extent of dissolution of synthetic apatites.

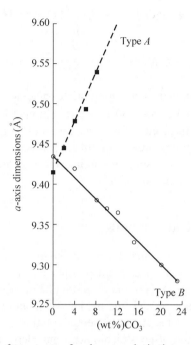

Figure 2.5 The effects of two types of carbonate substitution on the a-axis dimensions of synthetic apatites

2.2   Synthesis of Hydroxyapatite Powder

Hydroxyapatite (HA) powder [11 – 15] can be synthesized via numerous routes by using a range of different reactants under different processing conditions. The characteristics, such as morphology, stoichiometry, and level of crystallinity, of the HA powders vary by processing methods. According to the aqueous solvent usage, processing methods can be classified into two categories: dry and wet chemical methods.

2.2.1   Dry Chemical Methods

The solid-state reactions between calcium and phosphorus compounds are used in dry methods, which have the advantage of providing stoichiometric HA powders.

Pure HA powder can be prepared by solid-state reactions as follows:

$$6CaHPO_4 + 4Ca(OH)_2 \longrightarrow Ca_{10}(PO_4)_6(OH)_2 + 6H_2O$$

or

$$3Ca_3(PO_4)_2 + Ca(OH)_2 \longrightarrow Ca_{10}(PO_4)_6(OH)_2 + H_2O$$

The raw calcium compounds with appropriate ratio are milled, well mixed, compressed, and sintered above 950°C. A stoichiometric and well crystallized HA powder can be synthesized. However, this route requires a relatively high temperature and a long heat-treatment time. Moreover, sinterability of such powders is usually low. By using appropriate ratio of raw compounds, substituted apatites can be obtained as well.

2.2.2　Wet Chemical Methods

Either the precipitation from mixed aqueous solutions (chemical precipitation technique) or the hydrolysis of calcium phosphates can be used in wet routes, which have the advantages of producing more chemically reactive HA powders due to their high surface area and fine particle size, and low cost and simplicity owing to the use of supersaturated aqueous solutions. However, wet routes often lead to the formation of nonstoichiometric powders, the contamination with ions, such as carbonates, hydrogen phosphates, potassium, sodium, nitrates, and chloride, and the formation of deficient hydroxyapatites. All these uncontrollable variables may cause significant changes in their crystallographic characteristics. In general, nonstoichiometric HA obtained from aqueous solutions are mainly caused by the high chemical affinity of the apatites to these ions, the complex nature of the calcium phosphates system, and the kinetic and thermodynamic parameters, which highly depend on the experimental conditions. For instance, when synthesis of HA crystals from highly supersaturated solution, an intermediate precursor phase, such as tricalcium phosphate (TCP) and octacalcium phosphate, exists during synthesis process. Even after a prolonged time of reaction, traces of precursors can still be detected, which affect the stoichiometry of the final product.

　　The wet methods are used for the mass production of both crystalline HA and noncrystalline calcium phosphate powders. Two types of reaction are typically used in the wet method. One is a neutral reaction of acid and alkaline solutions, which was firstly developed by Tagai and Aoki, as follows:

$$10Ca(OH)_2 + 6H_3PO_4 \longrightarrow Ca_{10}(PO_4)_6(OH)_2 + 18H_2O$$

The other is a reaction of calcium salts and phosphate salts:

$$10CaCl_2 + 6Na_2HPO_4 + 2H_2O \longrightarrow Ca_{10}(PO_4)_6(OH)_2 + 12NaCl + 8HCl$$
$$10Ca(NO_3)_2 + 6(NH_4)_2HPO_4 + 2H_2O \longrightarrow$$
$$Ca_{10}(PO_4)_6(OH)_2 + 12NH_4NO_3 + 8HNO_3$$
$$6CaHPO_4 + 4Ca(OH)_2 \longrightarrow Ca_{10}(PO_4)_6(OH)_2 + 6H_2O$$
$$3Ca_3(PO_4)_2 + Ca(OH)_2 \longrightarrow Ca_{10}(PO_4)_6(OH)_2 + H_2O$$

Wet chemical methods include precipitation, hydrothermal techniques, hydrolysis of other calcium phosphates, etc.

2.2.2.1 Hydrothermal Reactions

The term hydrothermal usually refers to any heterogeneous reaction in the presence of aqueous solvents or mineralizes under high pressure and temperature conditions to dissolve and recrystallize materials that are relatively insoluble under ordinary conditions. Using this route, a high degree of crystallinity and a Ca : P ratio close to stoichiometric value can be obtained, because the intermediate precursor phase, such as β-TCP, $Ca_3(PO_4)_2$, tetracalcium phosphate (TTCP), $Ca_4P_2O_9$, and $Ca_4(PO_4)_2O$, can be easily converted to HA under hydrothermal condition.

The above reactions in solid-state reactions can also go through hydrothermally at 275 ℃, under steam pressure of 12,000 psi (1 psi = 0.070 kg/cm^2). The resulting HA is often carbonate substituted, but well crystallized and chemically homogenous. In order to avoid carbonate substitution, appropriate amounts of $CaHPO_4$ or $(NH_4)_2HPO_4$ can be added to the system to transform calcium carbonate to HA as follows:

$$4CaCO_3 + 6CaHPO_4 \longrightarrow Ca_{10}(PO_4)_6(OH)_2 + 6H_2O + 4CO_2$$

or

$$10CaCO_3 + 6(NH_4)_2HPO_4 \longrightarrow Ca_{10}(PO_4)_6(OH)_2 + 6NH_3 + 4H_2O + 10CO_2$$

2.2.2.2 Hydrolysis

HA powders can be obtained through the hydrolysis of other calcium phosphates. For example, many calcium phosphates, such as dicalcium phosphate dihydrate (DCPD), dicalcium phosphate anhydrous (DCP), tricalcium phosphate (TCP), amorphous calcium phosphate (ACP), octacalcium phosphate (OCP, $Ca_8H_2(PO_4)_6 \cdot 5H_2O$), calcium carbonate ($CaCO_3$), potassium phosphate carbonate, and so on, can be hydrolyzed to calcium-deficient hydroxyapatite powder. This approach is particularly attractive for several reasons. It only requires low temperatures, usually below 100°C for processing, increases the mechanical properties of calcium phosphates by hardening, utilizes a single precursor, and forms calcium-deficient HA which is more soluble than stoichiometric HA and therefore may be incorporated into bone more readily. For example, calcium-deficient HA can be formed as per the following reaction:

$$3Ca_3(PO_4)_2 + H_2O \longrightarrow Ca_9(HPO_4)(PO_4)_5OH$$

However, hydrolysis product is highly nonstoichiometric, and results in HA needles or blades with micron size range. Furthermore, the conventional hydrolysis at low temperature may take hours, even days to complete. Some scientists have combined with ultrasonic or microwave to speed up the hydrolysis process.

2.2.2.3 Precipitation Method

The preparation method is the most commonly used in commercial processing settings. A neutral reaction of acid, such as phosphoric acid (H_3PO_4), and alkaline solutions, such as calcium hydroxide ($Ca(OH)_2$), is often employed to obtain HA powders as shown below:

$$10Ca(OH)_2 + 3H_3(PO_4)_2 \longrightarrow Ca_{10}(PO_4)_6(OH)_2$$

This process can be modified by adding ammonium hydroxide ($NH_4(OH)$) to keep the pH of the reaction alkaline to insure the formation of HA after sintering the apatite precipitate.

A reaction between calcium nitrate ($Ca(NO_3)_2$) and ammonium phosphate ($(NH_4)_2HPO_4$) with added NH_4OH is also utilized to get HA powders as shown below:

$$10Ca(NO_3)_2 + 6(NH_4)_2HPO_4 + 2NH_4OH \longrightarrow$$
$$Ca_{10}(PO_4)_6(OH)_2 + 14NH_3 + 10H_2O + 20NO_2$$

Calcium acetate ($Ca(CH_3COO)_2$) is suggested to replace the use of calcium chloride or nitrate in precipitation reactions because the acetate ions will not be incorporated into the apatite, and nitrate or chloride ions may include into apatite.

The advantages with precipitation approach include low processing temperature, which ranges from room temperature (about 24°C) to boiling (95°C – 100°C), resulting nanometric-size crystals in blade, needle, rod, or equiaxed particle shape, usually leading to calcium deficient apatite, adjustable calcium concentration, and controllable substitutions in the products. For example, calcium can be replaced by many atoms, such as strontium, magnesium, manganese, etc. the phosphate can be substituted with carbonate, vanadate, borate, manganate, etc. and F-apatite or Cl-apatite can be obtained by adding F^- or Cl^- ions in the reaction.

However, the properties of HA powders, such as crystallinity and Ca : P ratio, are highly dependent on processing condition, such as the ratio and concentrations of the reactants and the pH of the reaction. Due to the presence of vacancies and ion substitutes in the lattice during the process, the HA powders are usually nonstoichiometry and low crystallinity.

In summary, pure HA powders can be obtained from many reactions either in hydrothermal systems or from solid-state reactions. However, when prepared from aqueous systems either by precipitation or hydrolysis methods, the apatite obtained is usually calcium deficient and HPO_4 enriched. Calcium phosphate reagents, such as $CaCO_3$, $Ca(OH)_2$, or CaO, can be used to correct calcium-deficient, if necessary. When the precipitation reaction is carried out under very basic conditions, the precipitation will contain carbonate, which will make the Ca : P molar ratio higher than the stoichiometric value. Other techniques have been used for making HA powders, such as electrocrystallization, emulsion, flux method, freeze drying, mechno-chemical method, microwave irradiation, plasma technique, sol-gel, spray-pyrolysis, and so on.

Thermal behavior of HA is one of the most concerning issues, because most ceramic processing is at high temperature. Interestingly, OH^- ions remain stable in the HA structure even at high temperatures ($\sim 1,350\,^{\circ}C$). This stability allows for high temperature processing.

2.3   Mechanical Properties of Hydroxyapatite

The value of the mechanical properties highly depends on the measurement techniques, and porosity, grain size and impurities of the HA samples. Therefore, most of the values presenting in this part are the ranges of the mechanical properties[16 − 20].

The Young's modulus data of dense HA materials are close to the hard tissue. For example, the Young's modulus is in the range of 35 − 120 GPa, and bending is in the range of 44 − 115 GPa, whereas the Young's modulus of hard tissue is in the range of 10 − 20 GPa. Bending strength, compressive strength and tensile strength of the dense HA are in the ranges of 38 − 250 MPa, 120 − 900 MPa, and 38 − 300 MPa, respectively, which are comparable to that of hard tissue. However, from the safety design of the biomedical implants point of view, the mechanical properties of dense HA are not good enough for most load-bearing applications. Moreover, HA materials have low values of K_{IC} and Weibull modulus (about $5-18$), which means that HA is a typical brittle ceramic, high susceptible to slow crack growth, and not reliable under load. For example, most of the loaded dental HA implants were broken within one year.

　　Generally, for dense HA materials, with the increase in Ca : P ratio, the strength increases, reaches the peak value around Ca : P = 1.67, and decreases abruptly when Ca : P > 1.67, as schematically shown in Fig.2.6.

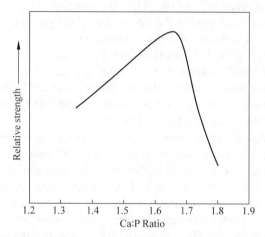

Figure 2.6 The effect of Ca : P ratio on the mechanical properties of HA materials

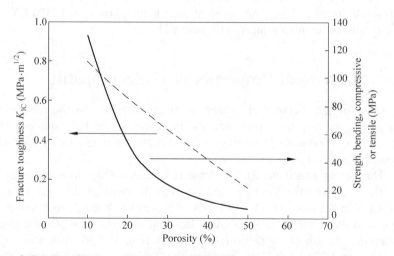

Figure 2.7 Schematic plots of fracture toughness (K_{IC}) and strength (bending, compressive and tensile) as a function of porosity of HA materials. (The values in this figure are relative.)

The mechanical properties of HA materials are affected strongly by the porosity of samples. For example, strength of HA samples decreases exponentially with the increasing porosity as schematically shown in Fig. 2. 7. Fracture toughness (K_{IC}) of dense HA is in the range of $0.8 - 1.2$ MPa $\cdot$ m$^{1/2}$, and it decreases almost linearly with increasing porosity, as shown schematically in Fig. 2. 7.

2.4　Other Bioceramics

2.4.1　Tricalcium Phosphate

Most investigations have demonstrated that the presence of HA is the key to form the osseointegration at the bioceramic-bone tissue interface. Moreover, the closer the solubility rate of bioceramics to the rate of bone tissue regeneration, the better bone tissue bonds with the bioceramics. Among all calcium phosphate bioceramics studied, stoichiometric HA is the one that dissolves and precipitates the slowest. From the dissolution and precipitation point of view, stoichiometric HA ceramic can be considered as a bioactive and nonbiodegradable bioceramics. As a result, tricalcium phosphate (TCP, $Ca_3(PO_4)_2$) has been developed as a bioactive and biodegradable bone substitute [21, 22].

A material with ideal biodegradability would be replaced by bone as it degraded. However, when used as a biomaterial for alveolar ridge augmentation, the rate of biodegradation of β-TCP has been shown to be too fast. To slow the rate of biodegradation, biphasic calcium phosphate (BCP) ceramics (i.e. composite ceramics that consist of mixtures of both the HA and β-TCP phases) have been used. β-TCP has a rhombohedral space group R3c. Its structure has one straight chain column [PO_4 — Ca $*$ — Ca_1 — PO_4 — Ca $*$ — Ca_2] with 0.5 probability of calcium, Ca $*$, and a zigzag chain column [PO_4 — Ca_3 — Ca_4 — Ca_5 — PO_4] $\cdot$ Ca $*$.

2.4.2　Bioactive Glasses

Except for calcium phosphate, another class of bioactive ceramics is bioactive glass [23, 24]. A potential advantage of bioactive glasses over HA and TCP is that it is possible to obtain a substrate from bioactive glass stronger than cortical bone and possess the ability to form a strong chemical bond with bone as well.

For example, a glass ceramic containing apatite and wollastonite was developed with better mechanical properties than bone tissue and with the ability to bond chemically with living bone tissue [25, 26]. Bioactive glasses are the glasses falling into the following compositional range: less than 60 mol % SiO_2, high Na_2O and CaO content, and a high $CaO:P_2O_5$ ratio. Bioactive glasses can be fabricated from a mixture of silica, alumina, magnesia, calcium oxide, sodium oxide, and phosphorous oxide. There are two types of bioactive glasses. One is silicate glasses, the other is calcium phosphate-based glasses (e.g. CaO-P_2O_5 glass). The bioactivity of bioactive glasses results from the formation of hydroxyapatite layer on the surface. When bioactive glass is exposed to tissue fluids, it forms a bonding layer of biological hydroxy-carbonate-apatite (HCA) on surface with an underlying layer of silica gel. Different calcium phosphates glasses exhibit widely different resorption properties. The resorption property of calcium phosphates depends on the $Ca:PO_4$ ratio, degree of crystallinity and crystal structure.

2.5   References

1. Schultz, O., et al. Emerging strategies of bone and joint repair. Arthritis Res. **2**(6): 433 −436 (2000)
2. Perry, C. R. Bone repair techniques, bone graft, and bone graft substitutes. Clin. Orthop. **360**: 71 −86 (1999)
3. Hamadouche, M., L. Sedel. Ceramics in orthopaedics. J. Bone Joint Surg. Br. **82**(8): 1095 −1099 (2000)
4. Bohner, M. Calcium orthophosphates in medicine: from ceramics to calcium phosphate cements. Injury. **31** Suppl 4 : 37 −47 (2000)
5. Ducheyne, P. Q. Qiu. Bioactive ceramics: the effect of surface reactivity on bone formation and bone cell function. Biomaterials. **20**(23 −24): 2287 −2303 (1999)
6. Burg, K. J., S. Porter, J. F. Kellam. Biomaterial developments for bone tissue engineering. Biomaterials. **21**(23): 2347 −2359 (2000)
7. Weiner, S., H. D. Wagner. The material bone: structure-mechanical function relations. Annual Review of Materials Science. **28**: 271 −298 (1998)
8. Deany, I. L. Recent advances in ceramics for dentistry. Crit. Rev. Oral. Biol. Med. **7**(2): 134 −143 (1996)
9. Gibson, I. R., S. M. Best, W. Bonfield. Chemical characterization of silicon-substituted hydroxyapatite. J. Biomed. Mater. Res. **44**(4): 422 −428 (1999)
10. Serre, C. M., et al. Influence of magnesium substitution on a collagen-apatite biomaterial on the production of a calcifying matrix by human osteoblasts. J. Biomed. Mater. Res. **42**(4): 626 −633 (1998)
11. Bouler, J. M., R. Z. LeGeros, G. Daculsi. Biphasic calcium phosphates: influence of three synthesis parameters on the HA/beta-TCP ratio. J. Biomed. Mater. Res. **51**(4):

680 − 684(2000)

12. El Briak-BenAbdeslam, H. E., et al. Dry mechanochemical synthesis of hydroxyapatites from dicalcium phosphate dihydrate and calcium oxide: a kinetic study. J. Biomed. Mater. Res. **67A**(3): 927 − 937 (2003)

13. Bourges, X., et al. Synthesis and general properties of silated-hydroxypropyl methylcellulose in prospect of biomedical use. Adv. Colloid. Interface. Sci. **99**(3): 215 − 228 (2002)

14. Ambrosio, A. M., et al. A novel amorphous calcium phosphate polymer ceramic for bone repair: I. Synthesis and characterization. J. Biomed. Mater. Res. **58**(3): 295 − 301(2001)

15. Kumar, T. S. S., I. Manjubala, J. Gunasekaran. Synthesis of carbonated calcium phosphate ceramics using microwave irradiation. Biomaterials. **21**(16): 1623 − 1629 (2000)

16. Yasuda, H. Y., et al. Microstructure and mechanical property of synthesized hydroxyapatite prepared by colloidal process. Biomaterials. **21**(20): 2045 − 2049 (2000)

17. Roeder, R. K., M. M. Sproul, C. H. Turner. Hydroxyapatite whiskers provide improved mechanical properties in reinforced polymer composites. J. Biomed. Mater. Res. **67A**(3): 801 − 812 (2003)

18. Werner, J., et al. Mechanical properties and in vitro cell compatibility of hydroxyapatite ceramics with graded pore structure. Biomaterials. **23**(21): 4285 − 4294 (2002)

19. Rodriguez-Lorenzo, L. M., et al. Hydroxyapatite ceramic bodies with tailored mechanical properties for different applications. J. Biomed. Mater. Res. **60**(1): 159 − 166 (2002)

20. Charriere, E., et al. Mechanical characterization of brushite and hydroxyapatite cements. Biomaterials **22**(21): 2937 − 2945 (2001)

21. Erbe, E. M., et al. Potential of an ultraporous beta-tricalcium phosphate synthetic cancellous bone void filler and bone marrow aspirate composite graft. Eur. Spine. J. **10** Suppl 2 : S141 − S146 (2001)

22. Metsger, D. S., T. D. Driskell, J. R. Paulsrud. Tricalcium phosphate ceramic—a resorbable bone implant: review and current status. J. Am. Dent. Assoc. **105**(6): 1035 − 1038 (1982)

23. Thompson, I. D., L. L. Hench. Mechanical properties of bioactive glasses, glass-ceramics and composites. Proc. Inst. Mech. Eng. **212**(2): 127 − 136 (1998)

24. Rawlings, R. D. Bioactive glasses and glass-ceramics. Clin. Mater. **14**(2): 155 − 179 (1993)

25. Sautier, J. M., et al. Bioactive glass-ceramic containing crystalline apatite and wollastonite initiates biomineralization in bone cell cultures. Calcif. Tissue Int. **55**(6): 458 − 466 (1994)

26. Ono, K., et al. Mechanical properties of bone after implantation of apatite-wollastonite containing glass ceramic-fibrin mixture. J. Biomed. Mater. Res. **24**(1): 47 − 63 (1990)

2.6 Problems

1. What is osseointegration and how is it achieved?
2. What is stress shielding?
3. What factors affect stress shielding?
4. The following Fig. 2.8 schematically shows the three types of loads on the femur implants. They are axial loads (i. e. the loads transmitted straight down the canal.), bending loads and torsional loads (i.e. the loads twisting around the long axis of the bone.). From the stress shielding point of view, which kind of loads are the most damaging?

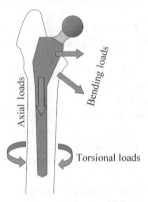

Figure 2.8 Implant loads

5. How do you study the properties of bioceramics coatings on the metal implants?
6. Why bioactive ceramics is coated on metal hard tissue implants?
7. What are the advantages of using bioactive ceramics for biomedical implants?
8. What is the major factors influencing the mechanical properties of hydroxyapatite?
9. What are the differences between the terms "ceramic" and "glass"?

3 Bioceramic Processing[*]

Bioceramics used as implants can take several forms, such as dense implant, porous network, micro-and nano-particle and sphere, coating, and composites with polymeric materials. Owing to the limited mechanical properties and superior bioactivity of bioceramics, and bioinertness and excellent mechanical strength of metallic biomaterials, bioceramic coating on metal implants is one very promising approach for orthopedic implants with both strength and bioactivity. Bioceramic coatings can provide stable fixation with tissue and shield the metal implants from corrosive environment. Previous studies have demonstrated that bioceramic coated metal implants form chemical bonds with bond tissue and allow for early functional loading. Moreover, the bioceramic coatings are not limited to metals. Bioceramic coatings can be applied on carbon, sintered ceramics, and polymers as well. The thickness of the bioceramic coatings varies from several microns to several hundreds microns. If the coating is too thick, it is easy to break. If the coating is too thin, it is easy to dissolve, because resorbability for HA, which is the slowest to dissolve in bioceramics, is about $15-30$ μm per year. Another problem with coatings is the delamination of the coating layer. In order to improve the bonding between the bioceramic coating and substrate, an intermediate layer consisting of Ca_2SiO_4 or bioactive glasses has been studied. In order to improve bone tissue fixation, a porous coating is desirable. Bioceramics are limited in their applications to only small, unloaded, and low-loaded implants, powders, coatings, composites, porous scaffolds for tissue engineering, and so on. We will focus on the bioceramic processing of porous substrate, micro- and nano- particle and sphere, coating, and composites in this chapter.

---

[*]   Authers are Donglu Shi and Xuejun Wen.

3.1 Fabrication and Mechanical Properties of Porous Bioceramics

Porous bioceramics, such as hydroxyapatite (HA), tricalcium phosphate (TCP) and bioactive glass, have been developed for hard tissue implants and tissue engineering scaffolds, owing to their excellent biocompatibility, bioactivity, and bioresorption in calcified tissue. Furthermore, porous substrates offer many advantages for hard tissue replacements. For example, porous substrates mimic the natural bone structure, which consists of 55% − 70% interconnected poro-sity, and would promote the osseointegration process; pores provide mechanic interlock that is good for implant fixation and early integration; porous structure provides a large surface area to volume ratio and therefore more contact surface for tissue bonding; an interconnected porous system would allow for cell and tissue intergrowth, nutrient and waste products transport, and a new blood vessel network formation. To fulfill the requirement for bone tissue integration, the main morphological requirements for the porous substrates are the existence of open and interconnected pores, with pore diameters larger than 100 μm for proper vascularization. There are two routes to fabricate three-dimensional porous substrates, which vary according to the temperature applied.

3.1.1 High Temperature Routes

3.1.1.1 Pyrolysis of Organic Particles

This method is adopted from a traditional ceramic processing. This method for fabricating highly porous bioceramic substitutes consists of four steps. The first step is the mixing of bioceramic raw powders with polymeric fillers. The polymeric fillers must be burned out completely leaving behind only non-toxic gases, such as polyvinyl butyral (PVB), starch, polystyrene, polymethyl metacrylate (PMMA). The appropriate amount, size, and shape of the polymeric fillers determine the three-dimensional architecture, macrostructure, and microstructure of the scaffolds. The second step is the compressing of the mixture into the desired shape under pressure. The third step is burning out of the polymer at a certain temperature for a particular time period. The final step is the sintering of the ceramic powders into porous solid form. Through this route, porosity of up to 70% can be obtained. However, the major problem with this method is that with the increasing porosity, the mechanical properties decrease dramatically. By combining this method with hot isostatic processing (HIP) and nanotechnology, the mechanical properties of the porous ceramics substrate may be improved to some extent. Even with these modifications, porous bioceramics are still not strong enough for load-bearing situations, owing to the brittle nature of the bioceramics.

3.1.1.2 Foam Sintering

This is one widely used process based on gas volatilization. Bioceramic powders are well mixed with naphthalene particles or hydrogen peroxide. The desirable shape is formed with isostatic compaction. Then the green body is subject to high temperature sintering. Additive particles or liquids are volatized and an isolated porosity, which consists of spherical voids communicated by a narrow neck, is obtained.

3.1.1.3 Gel-Casting

A polymer binder, e.g. methyl cellulose or polyethyleneimine, is used to mix with bioceramic powders to form a gel with proper viscosity. The gel is cast into a mold with the desired shape and thickness and is dried at $50\,^{\circ}C - 90\,^{\circ}C$. Then the green body is heated slowly to sintering temperature to form porous substrate.

3.1.1.4 Polymeric Sponge Technique

It is based on a replication concept. A polymeric sponge or foam, e.g. polyurethane or cellulose, is used as a template. Slurry of bioceramics impregnate the sponge, and the compound is subject to sintering to form porous substrate. However, the porous substrates fabricated using this approach possess low strength and fracture toughness; owing to the very thin ceramic, struts remain after the polymer is burned out.

3.1.1.5 Coextrusion Process

This technique may be used to fabricate macrochannelled HA substrates. HA powders are employed as starting materials, carbon black powders are used as fillers for macrochannel creation, and organic binders are used to glue the powders together. The organic binders must be burned out completely leaving behind only non-toxic gases, such as methyl cellulose, polyethyleneimine, ethylene ethyl acrylate (EEA) resin, or acryloid B67 resin. Briefly, by well mixing the HA powders with organic binders, and carbon black powders with organic binders, HA mixture is used as shell and carbon black is employed as channel core. At this stage, both the shell and the core are very big. The shell-core compound is then extruded several times to achieve thin shell and small core condition. The green body is subject to thermal treatment: Organic binder is burned out at about $500\,^{\circ}C - 700\,^{\circ}C$, and HA powders are sintered together at $1,200\,^{\circ}C - 1,350\,^{\circ}C$. The final step is the removal of the carbon black powders and the formation of macrochannelled substrates.

3.1.2 Low Temperature Routes

3.1.2.1 Leaching

Water-setting HA cements are needed to create HA substrates with various porosities using leaching technique. Water-setting HA cement bases on the reaction of precursors in an aqueous environment at room or body temperature, such as tetracalcium phosphate (TTCP) ($Ca_4(PO_4)_2$) and calcium hydrogen phosphate ($CaHPO_4$).

$$Ca_4(PO_4)_2 + CaHPO_4 \longrightarrow Ca_5(PO_4)_3OH$$

This HA cement sets in approximately 15 min and the isothermal chemical reaction is completed in about 4 h at $37\,^{\circ}C$. The pores are obtained by leaching approach. Sugar or salt particles are mixed with cement, and, after cement sets, particles are dissolved using water.

3.1.2.2 Hydrothermal Exchange

This process is firstly developed by Roy and Linnehan. It requires a relatively low temperature (e.g. $270\,^{\circ}C$), but very high pressure (e.g. 103 MPa), when compared with conventional high temperature route. In brief, it uses the skeletal structure of marine invertebrates, such as corals, as a template to make porous HA substrates. By a hydrothermal exchange of carbonate and phosphate using diammonium hydrogen phosphate (($NH_4)_2HPO_4$), the calcium carbonate skeleton can be converted to HA. The advantage of this process is that a nearly pure HA substrate with an interconnected porous structure, an exact replicate of the porous marine skeleton ($\sim 65\%$ porosity), can be obtained under suitable temperature and pressure.

3.1.2.3 Bicontinuous Microemulsion Technique

Using high temperature routes and other low temperature routes, only macro-porous ceramic substrates can be fabricated. Walsh developed a process called the bicontinuous microemulsion technique or crystal tectonics, which allows for the fabrication of porous scaffolds that are either mesoporous or macroporous. This technique is based upon the immiscibility phenomenon of emulsion like that used in emulsion freeze-drying techniques. Briefly, the scaffolds can be formed from oil-water-surfactant microemulsions supersaturated with biominerals. The pore size and structure are determined by the relative concentrations of water and oil. Since there is no report of using this material form as substrates for tissue replacements, further investigations on biocompatibility issues and cell behavior on these surfaces needs to be done. Such complex, three-dimensional architectures with either mesoporous or macroporous structures may be utilized as biomedical implants and scaffolds for tissue engineering organs, such as bone, as well as for some other important applications such as light-weight ceramics, catalyst supports, and robust membranes for high-temperature separation technology.

3.1.3 Rapid Prototyping Techniques

Rapid prototyping (RP) techniques, especially stereo lithography, are sophisti-cated techniques newly adopted in porous bioceramic scaffold fabrication. The three-dimensional bony defect that needs to be reconstructed can be obtained from a digital file of computer-aided design (CAD) or any imaging source, such as computer-tomography (CT) and nuclear magnetic resonance imaging (NMRI). The data can be used to fabricate three-dimensional objects through computer-aided fabrication (CAM) techniques. RP technology can be viewed as a three-dimensional printer. The prototype is created using a computer and the data can be transferred to the three-dimensional printer, which "prints" out the designed structure. This is especially advantageous when designing compli-cated objects. For example, the designed structure can be formed by curing a liquid resin and bioceramic mixture using laser radiation (photopolymerisation) and the very fine detail green body may be obtained. The green body can be directly used for implantation or followed up with a high temperature process-ing.

3.1.4 Mechanical Properties of Porous Bioceramics

Mechanical properties porous bioceramics highly depend on the degree of porosity, the distribution and the orientation of pores. For example, coralline HA shows apparent anisotropy, i.e. mechanical properties differ in one direction than in the others, as a result of the growth characteristics of most corals.

Mechanical properties of porous ceramic grafts increase with the bone tissue ingrowth. As mentioned earlier, tissue response to porous bioceramics differs from that of dense bioceramics owing to the tissue ingrowth possibility into porous implants. Porosity and interconnectivity are key determinants of the amount and type of ingrowth. Vigorous bone tissue ingrowth leads to the formation of a tissue-bioceramic composite with significantly improved mechanical properties. For example, the compressive strength increased 3 to 7 folds and anisotropy of the original substrate neutralized after bone tissue growth into the porous substrates. Moreover, a high correlation was found between the bending strength of porous HA and the amount of pore space occupied by bone tissue.

Porous bioceramics can be used for many applications including bone substitution (e.g. coatings on metal screws, pins and plates, powder/bulk bone fillings, etc.), scaffolds for tissue engineering application, soft tissue implants (e.g. orbital implants), and drug delivery devices. However, the major problem with porous bioceramics is their extremely poor mechanical properties, which are much lower than those of natural bone. Therefore, the future challenge is developing technology to produce highly porous bioactive substrates with superior mechanical properties.

3.2 Coating of Bioceramic Thick Films on Bio-Inert Porous Substrates

HA alone is not suitable for load bearing applications due to lower mechanical strength of HA. For load bearing applications, implants of bio-inert materials such as titanium, stainless steel, and titanium-vanadium alloys are used. These materials are generally coated with hydroxyapatite or bioactive glass for improving the biocompatibility and tissue growth surrounding them. The coating of HA films has been attempted on bio-inert materials of strength and/or toughness such as alumina, zirconia ceramics, titanium metal and titanium carbide. In evaluating HA coating methods, two factors are of primary importance. The first is whether the composition and properties of the coating are altered so that the *in vivo* performance of the coating is compromised. The second is that the coating should be strongly bonded to the substrate to maintain implant integrity as well to facilitate proper transmission of load from the implant to the surrounding bone. Many studies have demonstrated that bioceramic coatings can increase bone ingrowth when compared with non-coated bio-inert porous ceramic substrates and non-coated porous metal substrates. However, the level of the bone tissue ingrowth and bonding with the substrates varied greatly among these studies. The variation of the results may cause the differences in animal model used, Ca : P ratio, structural and compositional ceramic coatings, and pore size, pore morphology and properties of the porous substrate.

3.2.1 Slip Casting

Slip casting is a method for powder-based shaping of ceramic components that has been used for a long time in the traditional ceramic industry. Slip casting can be used for coating porous substrates as well. Slip casting is a filtration process, in which the porous substrates are dipped into a powder suspension for certain time and removed from the suspension. Owing to the capillary forces, liquid is sucked from the suspension (slip), and the powder particles are forced towards the walls of the pores and a consolidated layer is gradually built up. By properly controlling the dipping time, a desirable layer thickness can be obtained. After a certain period of drying the substrate then can be sintered for strong bonding. The advantages of slip casting as a forming method are that complex interconnected pores can be homogenously coated [1].

3.2.2 Electrophoretic Deposition

Electrophoretic deposition is a very effective and low cost technique for coating HA on porous substrates[2, 3]. During the process, fine HA powders are mixed in a liquid to form colloid at a desired pH value. By applying a constant current HA powders can be coated on metal substrates. This is a method which deposits the HA on an implant surface with minimal alteration of the starting material. However, as the HA is only weakly deposited and the individual particles are not bonded together, high temperature sintering is necessary after deposition. This is a useful technique for placing HA on porous metal surfaces that cannot be completely coated with line-of-sight techniques such as plasma spraying. To achieve a thick coating without defects, repeated deposition could be used instead of a single deposition. The green body is then dried before sintering.

3.2.3 Bioceramic-Glass Slurry Method

Using the bioceramic-glass slurry method [4], the substrates are first coated with a suspension containing the bioceramic powders followed by a sintering with an appropriate time-temperature cycle to densify the bioceramic coating. The flow chart of coating procedure is illustrated in Fig. 3.1. The coating suspension is made up of finely milled ceramic powders, an organic solvent, and a binder. The binder is used to prevent the precipitation of particles and to provide bonding strength to the coating after drying. One important property of the suspension is its viscosity. Specifically, when the porous substrate is immersed in the coating suspension, the suspension must be fluid enough to enter, fill, and uniformly coat the substrate skeleton. Low viscosity could result in undesirable thin films while highly viscous slurry would block the pore, thus impairing the interconnectivity of the pores. The viscosity is controlled by the relative amount of solvent, binder, and particles. The porous substrates are subsequently immersed into the mixture. After the porous substrates are completely infiltrated, they are spun briefly in a high-speed centrifuge to remove excess solution. Coated substrates are dried in an oven at $100\,^{\circ}C$. The dried specimens are heated in air to $400\,^{\circ}C$ for 1 h to burn out the organic binder from suspension. During the burnout process, a slow and controlled heating rate is necessary to avoid bubbling in the coating. Then the samples are subject to sintering at different temperatures. The slurry is prepared by suspending bioceramic particles and glass frits in an organic binder-solvent system. To coat HA on porous

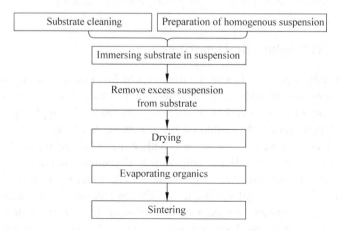

Figure 3.1 Flow chart of HA-glass slurry coating technique

Al_2O_3 substrate, the glass frits used are borosilicate glasses containing about 75% of a mixture of SiO_2 and B_2O_3 and 20 wt% alkali metal oxides. After melting, the glass is quenched in water and ground in a ball mill into a glass frit of the desired particle size. The coats developed by this method have a good adhesion to the Al_2O_3 substrate and weak reaction with HA during firing.

3.2.4 Thermal Deposition

Thermal deposition(TD) is a synthesis route [5,6]. In brief, by mixing calcium 2-ethyl hexanoate with bis(2-ethyhexyl) phosphite stoichiometrically in ethanol to form a homogenous suspension, the porous substrates are then subsequently immersed into the mixture. After the porous substrates are completely infiltrated, they are spun briefly in a high-speed centrifuge to remove the excess solution. Coated substrates are dried in an oven. The dried specimens are heated up to synthesize HA from precursors. The viscosity of the solution was controlled by the quantity of ethanol added. Then the samples were subject to sintering at different temperatures.

3.2.5 Sol-Gel Synthesis

A sol is a dispersion of colloidal particles, with diameter less than 100 nm, in liquid, and a gel is a three-dimensional, interconnected network formed from liquid. Sol-gel, being a rapidly advancing technology, is a low-temperature route for the synthesis and coating of ceramics, glasses, glass ceramics, and composites based on chemical solution reaction [7,8]. Sol-gel approach offers adjustable composition for bioceramics. According to the differences in gel formation and the processing temperature and pressure, sol-gel processes can be classified into three subtypes: gelation of colloidal powders, hypercritical drying, and hydrolysis and condensation of metal alkoxide precursors. In gelation, a gel is formed from colloidal particles through changing the pH of a sol. In hypercritical drying and hydrolysis and condensation of metal alkoxide precursors, a gel is formed from hydrolysis and condensation. Hydrolysis and condensation of metal alkoxide precursors occurs at ambient temperature and pressure, however, hypercritical drying is at elevated temperature and pressure.

The characteristics of sol-gel processing prove particular opportunities for synthesizing films in many applications. These include: (1) the solution employed can be vehicles for incorporating specific active constituents; (2) the highly porous intermediate state can be used to good advantage, and in providing contrast in properties between densified and non-densified regions; (3) the ease of changing composition makes available a wide range of chemical reactivity; (4) the range of properties between the just deposited gel and final glass opens a useful window in mechanical properties which permit procedures such as embossing to be applied to coatings; (5) in the case of multicomponent coatings, problems with vapor phase deposition methods (use of multiple targets, preferentially deposition of specific components, etc.) are substantially reduced or eliminated, and (6) the ability to coat large areas and non-flat geometries with economic efficiency.

Formation of the films on various substrates via the sol-gel process can be done by several solution deposition techniques. They include dip — coating, spin coating, spray coating, roller coating, and meniscus coating. Dip coating can be used to prepare the first sol-gel coatings many years ago to produce architectural windows up to 4 m × 5 m in size. Spin coating owes much of its development to the microelectronics industry where it has proved to be a rapid and efficient method of coating silicon wafers. It is also, within limitations, a quick and convenient method for the preparation of sol-gel coatings. Meniscus or laminar film coating is a comparatively new method that has shown some promise for the preparation of sol-gel optical coatings particularly on large square or rectangular substrates. Whereas dip coating, for example, can be used for samples of almost any shape or size, spin coating is easier if samples are round and comparatively small, and meniscus coating if samples are square or rectangular and comparatively large. Samples for meniscus coating must also be flat.

A wide range of compositions can be synthesized using sol-gel approach, and doping can readily be effected. The sol-gel technique offers a low-temperature method for synthesizing materials that are either totally inorganic in nature or composed of inorganic and organic. The process is based on hydrolysis and condensation reactions of organometallic compounds in alcoholic solutions. Films formed using sol-gel techniques represent the oldest commercial application of sol-gel technology. Today, sol-gel film coatings are being intensively studied for such diverse applications as protective and optical coatings, passivation and planarization layers, sensors, high or low dielectric constant films, inorganic membranes, electrooptic and non-linear optical films, electrochromics, strengthening layers, and ferroelectrics.

A sol-gel solution can be formed from an array of discrete colloidal particles by changing the pH value of the solution, or from the hydrolysis and condensation of liquid metal-alkoxide precursors. The substrates, including glass, alumina and silicon are usually dip-coated or spin-coated with the sol-gel solution. As the hydrolysis syntheses are performed under rather tractable conditions, HA with various Ca : P ratios are easily obtained. Another advantage of this method is that it can be applied to a substrate having complicated shape, like porous substrate.

The sol-gel process uses inorganic or metal organic precursors. The most commonly used organic precursors for sol-gel film formation are metal alkoxides ($M(OR)_z$), where R stands for an alkyl group (C_xH_{2x+1}). Normally, the alkoxide is dissolved in alcohol and hydrolyzed by adding water under acidic, neutral or basic conditions, although film formation is also possible by depositing alkoxides followed by exposure to moisture.

3.2.6 Biomimetic Growth

The bioceramic coatings can grow on the substrate surface [9], such as Ti, alumina, silica and polymer surface, in simulated body fluid at physiological conditions. The formed films are very uniform and dense. However, the growth rate is somewhat slow, only several micrometers per day. In brief, porous substrates are soaked into simulated body fluids and Ca − P layers are deposited on their surface under modulated nucleation and crystal growth conditions. A two-step procedure is developed; after the substrates are cleaned, they are pretreated in a solution containing inorganic components in the concentration more or less similar to body fluid and a thin amorphous carbonated Ca − P layer precipiated on the substrates. Second, by soaking these thinly coated substrates in another fluid with different concentrations, the thin Ca − P layer led to the fast precipitation of a second and thick Ca − P layer. In contrast to other coating approach, a number of bioactive Ca − P phases, such as octacalcium phosphate and B-carbonated apatite, participating normal bone tissue formation can be achieved using this approach.

3.3 Coating on Dense Substrates

All the coatings methods mentioned earlier can be used for coating on dense substrate.

3.3.1 Enameling

Enameling is a technique involving the firing of glass onto metal substrates [10]. Enameling procedure is very simple and a micron-sized thick layer of bioceramics can be coated on metal implants. Coated layers can be fine-tuned at the metal-glass and glass-bone interfaces so that the coating binds with both metal and bone. Bioactive glasses are used to obtain the same thermal expansion coefficient as the substrate metal implants and avoid the generation of thermal stresses at the interface. In order to obtain both strong and compatible interface and bioactivity of the coating, several layers of bioceramics are coated.

3.3.2 Plasma-Sprayed Coatings

This is the most common means of applying HA coatings to implant devices, employs a plasma, or ionized gas, partially to melt and carry the ceramic particulate onto the surface of the substrate, including atmospheric plasma spraying, vacuum plasma spraying and high-velocity oxy-fuel spraying (HVOF) [11,12]. In brief, particulate materials are injected into the high temperature heat sources where they are melted and propelled at high velocity towards a substrate. The molten droplets flatten on impact as splats to form a lamellar coating structure on the substrates. The advantages of plasma spraying for HA coatings include simplicity, high deposition rate, low substrate temperature, variable coating porosity, and variable phase and structure. Although plasma spraying is conceptually a simple process, there are many problems associated with this technique. The very high temperature of plasma spraying can lead to dehydroxylation or phase transformations in the coating. Plasma spraying also decreases crystallinity. An important aspect of plasma sprayed ceramic coatings is their thickness: mismatch in thermal properties coupled with the fast coating rate of the coating material during the plasma spray process gives rise to stresses in the coating and substrates; these stresses increase with the thickness of the coating. The compressive stress at the coating-substrate interface weakens the bond strength. Therefore, the thinner the coating, the higher its bond strength. Lack of consistency and reliability of HA coatings are major concerns on plasma spraying techniques. Investigations have shown that there are over 100 variables in the process influencing the coating characteristics. For example, variation in powder morphology can induce microstructural and mechanical inconsistencies that have an effect on the service performance of the coating [11].

Plasma-sprayed coatings of HA deposited onto medical and dental implants made of pure metals and alloys, for example, are widely used in reconstructive orthopaedic and dental surgery due to their excellent biocompatibility and bioactivity. However, the clinical usefulness, in terms of long-term stability, of such HA coatings has been questioned on the basis of reported loosening and subsequent failures of implanted prostheses. These failures mainly occur due to the degradation (both chemical and physical) and fatigue behaviors of these coatings. For example, a combination of aqueous environment and stress has been reported to cause delamination or accelerated dissolution of the coating. In particular, the adhesion strength of the coating to the implant surface appears to be a property that needs to be maximized to improve the implant fixation. The failure of implants leads to revision surgeries, which are expensive and compromise the lifestyle of patients.

To solve the above-mentioned problems, several new approaches and deposition techniques are being investigated for depositing stable, highly adhesive HA coatings onto implant materials. The incorporation of biocompatible bond coats such as titania for improving the interfacial adhesion between the plasma-sprayed HA coating and the implant surface is one such approach. The use of the radio frequency (RF) sputtering technique for the deposition of HA thin-film coatings is another approach that has gained significant momentum, primarily owing to the deposition advantages this technique possesses over other techniques. For example, RF sputtered HA coatings are more retentive and their structure (hence *in vivo* dissolution) can be precisely controlled. Sputtered HA can be applied to coat implants of complex shapes, and these coatings are very thin (a few microns in thickness) but provide complete substrate coverage and hence can be applied to fine implant structures such as threaded dental and craniofacial implants without compromising their essential design. HA by sputtering, being a vacuum-based process, can be easily and sequentially adapted for incorporating bond coats such as titania and silica for realizing composite implant/bond-coat/HA structures. In addition, sputtered HA coatings can also be deposited to have a graded microstructure for selective dissolution of the coating *in vivo*, that is, a sub-layer with high crystallinity (implying low dissolution rate) in immediate contact with the implant surface and an amorphous sub-layer (implying high dissolution rate) on the top. This type of graded HA layer is considered beneficial to the initial stages of implant fixation.

3.3.3 Sputtering

Ion beam sputtering and radio frequency sputtering are thin film deposition techniques in which a target material is bombarded with an ion beam in a vacuum chamber, and atomic sized fragments of sputtered material form coatings on suitably placed substrates. The typical coatings sputtered from a HA target are amorphous on deposition, as the sputtered components from the HA target (Ca, P, O and H) do not posses enough energy to recombine into HA. A heat treatment on the order of $500\,^{\circ}\text{C}$ is usually sufficient to provide enough thermal energy to form a crystalline coating, which is predominantly HA. Sputter deposited coatings generally have better bond strength and mechanical properties than thick coatings.

3.4 Hydroxyapatite Coatings for Non-Hard Tissue Applications

Metal stents have been used as an extremely effective solution to treat blood vessel stenosis. However, recurrence of blockage in the blood vessels (restenosis) often requires a repeat operation. To overcome restenosis problem, polymer coatings with/without drug eluting have been extensively studied. However, the body senses polymers as a foreign agent and some studies suggest this biochemical characteristic alone can trigger an inflammatory response leading to restenosis of the implanted stent. HA, a naturally existing material in body, can rapidly integrate into the host tissue, and is not recognized as a foreign agent. These beneficial factors may inhibit the inflammatory response mechanisms, which lead to restenosis. Therefore, porous HA could be a candidate coating on the surface of the stents. The thin coating (<500 nm), can be used as a "barrier" to prevent metal ion leaching as well. Additionally, HA shows great potential for drug eluting strategies. With the recent developments in micro-encapsulation technology, HA micro-spheres are being considered for drug delivery applications. HA has the advantage of being biocompatible, bioresorbable and highly binding to a variety of molecules (e.g. proteins, enzymes, antibody fragments, nucleic acids). This has opened the potential for using HA to deliver a large variety of drugs in many clinical applications. For this particular application, both sol-gel coating approach and radio frequency plasma coating method will work. The typical thickness of the coatings is summarized in Fig. 3.2.

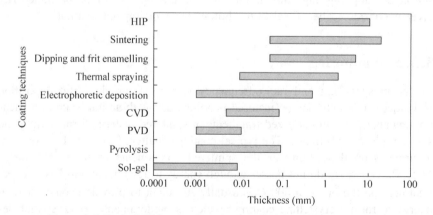

Figure 3.2 Typical thickness of coatings applied by different processes

3.5　Composites

Owing to the poor mechanical properties of bioceramics, many strategies have developed to improve the mechanical property; meanwhile to keep the bioactivity of the bioceramic. One example is the development of bioceramic-based composites.

3.5.1　Bioceramic-Polymer Composite

As discussed earlier in Chapter 2, the main chemical compositions of natural bone tissue are inorganic materials (e.g. calcium phosphate, ~ 70 wt%) and organic materials (e.g. collagen, 20 wt%). The calcium phosphate exists in the form of crystallized HA and amorphous calcium phosphate, and bonds with microfibril collagen. To mimic the chemical composition and structure of natural bone tissue, it is reasonable to develop composites consisting of both inorganic component and organic component.

HA-biodegradable polymer composites are developed with improved ductility and strength. The composites show a transition point. When HA percentage is lower than this point, the composites have the superior strength and toughness, and suitable Young's modulus for bone replacement. However, when HA percentage is over the point, the mechanical properties decrease abruptly. The composites have low bioactivity when compared with pure HA.

To more closely mimic the bone composition, HA-collagen composites are investigated. Although the composition of HA-collagen composites can be identical to natural bone, the complex microstructure cannot be achieved so far. There are at least three types of method used to fabricate the composites: high pressure molding method, UV irradiation, and precipitation of HA on collagen surfaces. By using high pressure molding method, HA-collagen composites were developed. However, the strength (e.g. compression strength is only about 6 – 10 MPa) is not strong enough for hard tissue replacement, although the elastic modulus, about 2 GPa, is slightly lower than the normal bone tissue. Moreover, the composite is not stable in an aqueous environment. Precipitation of HA crystals on collagen fibers is a very interesting way to mimic the bone formation during development. Although the mechanical property of HA-collagen composites is far from satisfaction, HA-collagen composites exhibit higher bioactivity in promoting bone regeneration than either HA or collagen alone.

HA in whisker form can be used as reinforcement phase in polymer-bioceramic composites. The interesting feature of using whisker is that the crystallographic orientation and in turn mechanical anisotropy similar to the natural bone may be obtained by controlling the size, aspect ratio, volume fraction, and preferred crystallographic orientation of the whiskers within a polymeric matrix, because mechanical anisotropy in human cortical bone is largely due to the alignment of bone mineral crystal. However, whisker form HA may have the risk of carcinogenic effect.

3.5.2 Reinforced Hydroxyapatite

Many reinforcements, for example, nano- and micro-particles, blades, whiskers, fibers, etc. made of metal, ceramic, and glass, have been employed to improve the mechanical properties, such as toughness and strength, of bioceramics. However, most reinforcements may lead to an increase of elastic modulus and a decrease of bioactivity. Moreover, if the metal is used as reinforcement phase, corrosion and metal ion release may cause negative tissue response. To avoid the decrease in bioactivity, bioactive glass reinforced HA composite is developed. Glass reinforced HA composite can be produced by mixing HA and bioactive glasses. The composite exhibits bioactivity and higher mechanical properties when compared to single phase HA. One example of glass reinforced HA composite is the composite consists of HA and a phosphate-based glasses (e.g. $CaO - P_2O_5$) glass. This process not only can improve the mechanical properties but also is able to increase the bioactivity of the substrate. For example, the composite of $CaO - P_2O_5$ glass reinforced HA is stronger than the pure HA through a transformation toughening mechanism. Furthermore, during the sintering process, the phosphate glass causes some of the HA to decompose to TCP, which is more bioactive than pure HA for promoting bone tissue regeneration. Through bioactive glass reinforcement, the strength, toughness, and density of the bioceramic are improved, and the bioactivity is kept. However, the material is still not strong enough for high loading applications. In order to fabricate porous structure, organic spheres, such as wax or polymer, can be added during the green body formation.

3.5.3 Hydroxyapatite and Tricalcium Phosphate Composite

Previous data suggest that the closer of the solubility rate of bioceramic to the rate of bone tissue regeneration, the better the bone tissue bonds with the bioceramics. Among all calcium phosphate bioceramics studied, stoichiometric HA is the one that dissolves and precipitates the slowest. From the dissolution and precipitation point of view, stoichiometric HA ceramic can be considered as a bioactive and nonbiodegradable bioceramic. As a result, tricalcium phosphate (TCP) has been developed as a bioactive and biodegradable bone substitute. However, the resorption rate of TCP is faster than bone tissue regeneration, because TCP may completely dissolve in days or weeks. Furthermore, TCP is mechanically much weaker than both HA and bone. Therefore, it may be advantageous to develop a composite from HA and TCP with a desirable resorption kinetics and better mechanical properties by varying the ratios of hydroxyapatite and tricalcium phosphate. The term "composite" is not appropriate for the mixture of HA and TCP here because they are in the same category of materials.

3.6　Summary

In summary, bioceramics have many biomedical applications including coatings for cementless implanted hip-joint, maxillofacial reconstruction, hard and soft tissue augmentation, otolaryngologyical implants, artificial tendons and ligaments, drug delivery carriers, etc. , due to their biocompatibility and highly bioactive nature. However, their poor mechanical performances limit their use in monolithic form in most load-bearing situations. Fortunately, the major advances in surface coating techniques and composite design are enabling their huge contribution in orthopedic applications. Presently, some new biomedical applications of dense HA are emerging, for example, dense HA materials have been used as percutaneous devices for continuous ambulatory peritoneal dialysis, monitoring of blood pressure and blood sugar, optical observation of inner body tissue, and so on.

3.7　References

1. Inoue, K., et al. Control of crystal orientation of hydroxyapatite by using a high magnetic field. Key Engineering Materials. **240 – 242**: 513 – 516(2003)
2. Wang, R., Y. X. Hu. Patterning hydroxyapatite biocoating by electrophoretic deposition. J. Biomed. Mater. Res. **67A**(1): 270 – 275(2003)
3. Ma, J., C. Wang, K. W. Peng. Electrophoretic deposition of porous hydroxyapatite scaffold. Biomaterials. **24**(20): 3505 – 3510(2003)
4. Jiang, G., D. Shi. Coating of hydroxyapatite on highly porous Al_2O_3 substrate for bone substitutes. J. Biomed Mater. Res. **43**(1): 77 – 81(1998)
5. Shi, D., G. Jiang, X. Wen. In vitro bioactive behavior of hydroxylapatite-coated porous $Al_{(2)}O_{(3)}$. J. Biomed. Mater. Res. **53**(5): 457 – 466(2000)

6. Jiang, G., D. Shi. Coating of hydroxyapatite on porous alumina substrate through a thermal decomposition method. J. Biomed. Mater. Res. **48**(2): 117 – 120(1999)
7. Hsieh, M. F., et al. Phase purity of sol-gel-derived hydroxyapatite ceramic. Biomaterials. **22**(19): 2601 – 2607(2001)
8. Liu, D. M., T. Troczynski, W. J. Tseng. Water-based sol-gel synthesis of hydroxyapatite: process development. Biomaterials. **22**(13): 1721 – 1730(2001)
9. Barrere, F., et al. Biomimetic calcium phosphate coatings on Ti_6AI_4V: a crystal growth study of octacalcium phosphate and inhibition by Mg^{2+} and HCO_{3-} Bone. **25**(2 Suppl): 107S – 111S(1999)
10. Gomez-Vega, J. M., et al. Bioactive glass coatings with hydroxyapatite and bioglass particles on Ti-based implants. 1. Processing. Biomaterials. **21**(2): 105 – 111(2000)
11. Cheang, P., K. A. Khor. Addressing processing problems associated with plasma spraying of hydroxyapatite coatings. Biomaterials **17**(5): 537 – 544(1996)
12. Sun, L., et al. Material fundamentals and clinical performance of plasma-sprayed hydroxyapatite coatings: a review. J. Biomed. Mater. Res. **58**(5): 570 – 592(2001)

3.8　Problems

1. Describe the generic procedures to fabricate porous bioceramics substrate using high temperature routs?
2. What is bicontinuous microemulsion technique?
3. What are the major factors influencing the mechanical property of porous bioceramics substrates? How does *in vivo* implantation affect their mechanical property?
4. Compare the methods for coatings on porous substrate in terms of coating thickness, chemical structure, mechanical property, and processing parameters.

4 Coating of Hydroxyapatite onto Inner Pore Surfaces of the Reticulated Alumina *

4.1 Hydroxyapatite Coating Methods and Characterization

4.1.1 Coating of Hydroxyapatite by the Hydroxyapatite-Glass Slurry Method

There have been various methods developed to produce Hydroxyapatite(HA) coatings [1 – 4]. Among these techniques, plasma spraying has widely been used [3]. This method is not, however, applicable for depositing HA films on a porous substrate. A suspension method has, therefore, been employed in the present investigation. It should be noted that such a method has been previously applied only on dense zirconia and titanium alloy [4] substrates. In this method, ceramic substrates are first coated with a suspension containing the HA powder. It is then sintered at an appropriate time-temperature cycle to densify the HA coating. Various experimental techniques have been used to characterize the coated product. Particular attention has been drawn to the microstructure, mechanical properties, and bonding behavior at the interface between the coating and the substrate.

The flowchart for the coating procedure is shown in Fig. 4.1. Two types of suspension were developed for coating. Solution A is prepared by suspending HA particles (~300 mesh) (Chemat Technology, Inc.) in an organic binder-solvent system. In solution B, HA was partially substituted by glass frits (65 wt%), which have good adhesion to the Al_2O_3 substrate and weak reaction with HA during firing. The glass frits used in this work were borosilicate glasses, containing about 75 wt% of a mixture of SiO_2, B_2O_3 and 20 wt% alkali metal oxides Na_2O. After melting, the glass was quenched in water and

---

∗ Authors are Donglu Shi and Gengwei Jiang.

ground in a ball mill into a glass frit of the desired particle size (~ 325 mesh).

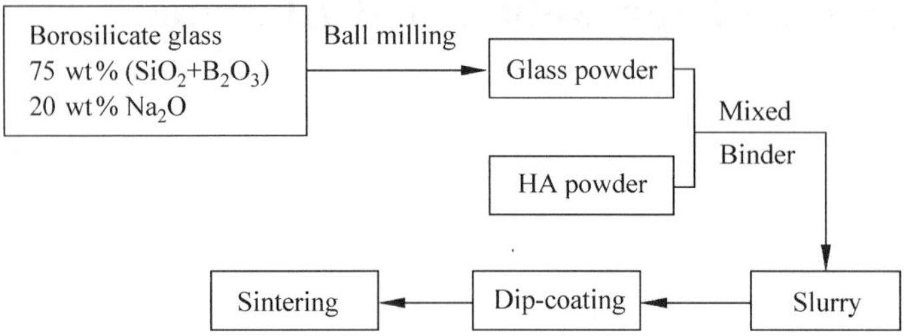

| Borosilicate glass 75 wt% ($SiO_2+B_2O_3$) 20 wt% Na_2O | Ball milling → Glass powder |
| HA powder | Mixed Binder |
| Sintering ← Dip-coating ← Slurry |

Figure 4.1 Flowchart of coating technique

Reticulated alumina (Al_2O_3) was used as the substrate material. Figure 4.2 is the cross-section of the reticulated alumina showing the interconnectivity of the pores in its structure. The size of the interconnected pores was large enough to allow the ingrowth of bone tissue. A HA ceramic layer was coated on both the outer and inner surface of the substrates. For the convenience of characterizing the coating properties, dense alumina plates were also coated using the conventional dip-coating method [4]. These substrates were cleaned in acetone and dried at $100°C$. They were subsequently immersed into the suspension. After the porous specimens were completely infiltrated, they were spun

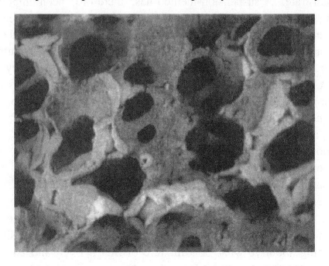

Figure 4.2 Cross-section of reticulated alumina substrate, showing the interconnected porosity

briefly in a high-speed centrifuge to remove excess solution. Coated substrates were dried in an air oven at 100°C. The dried specimens were heated in air to 400°C for 1 h to burn out the organic binder from the suspension. A slow and controlled heating rate was necessary to avoid bubbling in the coating. The coatings were calcined at a temperature of 900°C for 30 min. The coatings made from solutions A and B was further subjected to a heat treatment of 1,500°C for 3 h and 1,000°C for 30 min respectively. After the final heat treatment, strongly bonded HA thin films had been coated onto these substrates.

Although the slurry method is applicable for porous substrates, the major concern with this method is the biological stability of the glass, which serves as a sintering aid in the coating. Another problem associated with this method is the difficulty in preparing the well-dispersed suspension.

The phase diagram for anhydrous calcium phosphates (Fig. 4.3) shows that the liquid phase appears at a temperature above 1,500°C; and presumably the induced liquid could improve the bonding between HA and the Al_2O_3 substrate during sintering. However, such a liquid-enhanced bonding process was not experimentally observed. X-ray diffraction(XRD) analysis of the coating made from solution A showed that HA was decomposed, and in turn, the bioactivity of the coating would be changed. A high density of cracks was found to exist in the coating. The adherence of the coating to the Al_2O_3 substrates

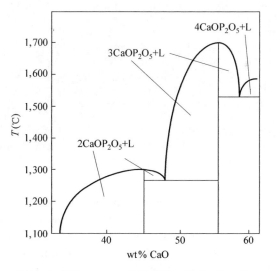

Figure 4.3 Phase diagram of the system $CaO-P_2O_5$, indicating the appearances of the liquid phase at high temperatures

was low and the ceramic layer could be peeled off by scraping. These results indicated that solution A was not suitable for this particular application.

Using the glass as a sintering aid, a well-bonded HA coating was produced. Figures 4.4 through Fig. 4.6 are scanning electron microscope (SEM) photographs of the surfaces and interfaces of the coatings made from solution B. As is apparent from Fig. 4.4 and Fig. 4.5, the glass-HA ceramic layer is firmly attached to the alumina substrate. An average coating thickness is 5 μm. The interfacial strength between the coating and the substrate depended on the adherence of the glass to the Al_2O_3. Figure 4.7 is the aluminum compositional profile across the interface. The data showed that the aluminum concentration decreased when scanning from the substrate to the outer surface of the coating. It was concluded that aluminum ions diffused during sintering, and consequently bonded the glass to the alumina substrate by ion diffusion. This diffusion bonding is probably attributed to the formation of a eutectic compound at the interface during the sintering, and thus ensures the strong bonding between the coating and the substrate. Further investigations of bonding and sintering mechanisms are underway.

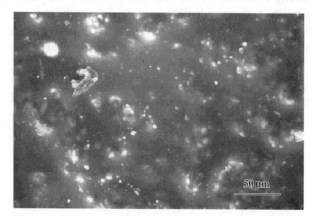

Figure 4.4 SEM photograph showing the HA-coated surface

From the above results, we see that the development of glass frits having an excellent adhesion to the alumina substrate were essential for producing the HA coating. Great efforts have therefore been made in the preparation of the glass frits. As a sintering aid, the glass must be wetting to the substrate and HA, and its melting point should be lower than the decomposing temperature of HA ($1,300°C$). Furthermore, for successful coating, optimizing the coefficient of thermal expansion of the glass to match the substrate is critical. It has been known that the mismatch in expansion coefficients between the coating

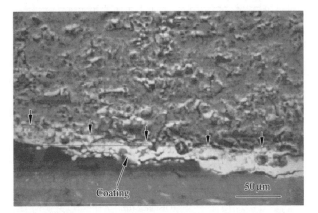

Figure 4.5 SEM photograph showing the HA-coating interface for dense alumina. The interface is indicated by arrows

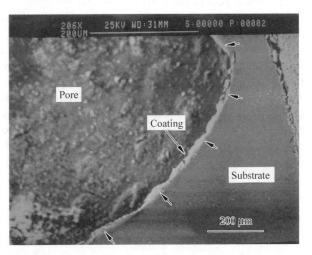

Figure 4.6 SEM photograph showing the HA-coating for porous alumina. As indicated by the arrows, a thin HA layer is uniformly coated onto the inner pore surface

and the substrate materials will give rise to interfacial stress which weakens the bond strength, or leads to the cracking of the coating. The magnitude of this stress is proportional to the difference between the thermal expansion coefficients of the coating and the substrate. The expansion coefficient of HA ($13.3 \times 10^{-6}/°C$) is relatively higher than that of alumina ($8.0 \times 10^{-6}/°C$). The expansion coefficient of the selected glass should then be an intermediate one to reduce this difference.

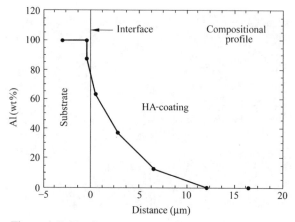

Figure 4. 7 Aluminum content profile across the interface

Another important aspect of the glass is chemical durability. For biological applications, it is essential for glass to be non-toxic and stable in the body fluid (BF). The dissolution of the glass will lead to the degradation of the coating. HA particles will escape from the coating, and this will have an extremely negative effect on the bone regeneration, such as interfacial loosening and tissue inflammation.

The optimal properties of the glass can be achieved by adjusting the glass compositions. The glass selected in this work is borosilicate glass. Its expansion coefficient is compatible with that of Al_2O_3 substrate. No crack was found in the coating (Fig. 4. 4). X-ray diffraction (XRD) pattern of the coating (Fig. 4. 8) shows that there is no negative reaction between the glass and HA.

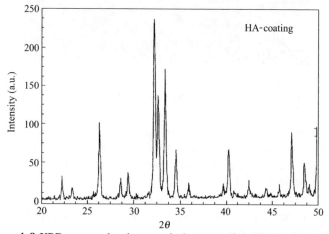

Figure 4. 8 XRD spectra showing a typical pattern of the HA-coating surface

Figure 4. 8 is a typical HA diffraction pattern. The *in vitro* experiments are currently being performed to investigate its biological stability.

4.1.2 Coating of Hydroxyapatite by a Thermal Deposition Method

In the so-called thermal deposition (TD) method, we completely remove the glass phases that could be potentially toxic. In TD, calcium 2-ethyl hexanoate was mixed with Bis(2-ethyhexyl) phosphite stoichiometrically in ethanol. The viscosity of the solution was controlled by the quantity of ethanol added. The mixture was stirred for 2 days at room temperature. The solution was used for coating both dense and porous alumina. The coating method was described previously [1]. Coated substrates were then air dried and calcinated up to $1,000\,^{\circ}C$ at a heating rate of $2\,^{\circ}C/min$. For phase analysis, the HA was also prepared in powder form. The solution was open to the air and stirred to vaporize the solvent. Finally, a highly viscous, translucent mixture was obtained. It was subsequently calcinated at the desired temperatures in air.

The suspension was basically made up of finely divided ceramic particles, an organic solvent and binder. The binder was used to prevent the precipitation of particles and to provide bonding strength to the coating after drying. One important property of the suspension is its viscosity. Specifically, when the porous substrate was immersed in the suspension, the suspension must be fluid enough to enter, fill, and uniformly coat the substrate skeleton. Low viscosity could result in undesirably thin films while highly viscous slurry would block the pore, thus damaging the interconnectivity of the pores. The viscosity was controlled by the relative amount of solvent, binder and particles.

4.1.3 Characterization of Hydroxyapatite Film

Fourier transform infrared spectroscopy (FTIR) was used to determine the reaction chemistry of the coated HA after firing. Figure 4.9 shows FTIR of unfired sample and samples fired at $500\,^{\circ}C$, $600\,^{\circ}C$, $700\,^{\circ}C$ and $900\,^{\circ}C$. According to standard IR transmission spectra, peaks observed at $3,573\ cm^{-1}$ and $631\ cm^{-1}$ are assigned to OH stretching and librational modes. Peaks around $600\ cm^{-1}$ and $1,100\ cm^{-1}$ are due to bending and stretching modes of $P-O$ bonds in phosphate groups. These are characteristic peaks of HA. At a sintering temperature of $500\,^{\circ}C$, $P-O$ bonds have formed, but hydroxyl groups were not detected. Comparing the spectra of unfired sample, most organic groups were burned out by this temperature. At $600\,^{\circ}C$, all the characteristic lines of HA were recorded, but some organic residual could still be seen. From 700°C and higher, the peak positions match all those of standard HA, and the organic groups were not detectable.

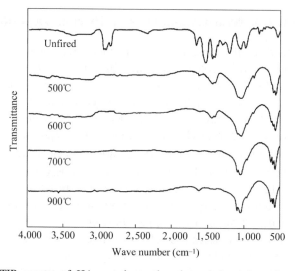

Figure 4.9 FTIR spectra of HA-coated samples sintered for 4 h at the temperatures indicated

Figure 4.10 are XRD spectra of HA sintered at different temperatures in the range of 600°C to 900°C. The results of X-ray diffraction(XRD) are quite consistent with that of FTIR. Crystalline phase started to form at 600°C, and all peaks were attributed to the HA phase. According to the Scherer equation:

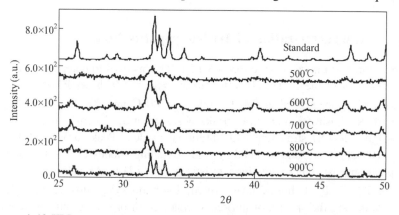

Figure 4.10 XRD spectra of HA-coated samples sintered for 4 h at the temperatures indicated. Note that the top spectrum is for the standard HA

$\Delta(2\theta) = 0.9\lambda/D$, where θ is differention angle, λ is wavelength and D is crystal size. The crystal size is inversely proportional to the peak width. The broadening of peaks was evident at lower sintering temperatures, indicating the initial state of crystal formation. At higher sintering temperatures, the growth of crystal was evidenced by the sharpening of peaks. The peak shift could also be noted by comparing with the standard XRD spectra of HA. At lower temperatures, the shift was considerable, suggesting great lattice distortion.

To monitor the sintering process and the evolution of chemical bonds is important in determining the bioactivity of the sintered products. The material with more lattice defects would be expected to be more reactive. This assumption will be verified experimentally later in *in vitro* tests. The high temperature and long time sintering will result in well-crystallized products. Therefore, to enhance the bioactivity, the low temperature and short time sintering is preferred. It is critical to find an optimal sintering procedure so that the sintered HA are poorly crystallized but with no organic residuals. The differential thermal analysis (DTA) profile (Fig. 4.11) shows that burn out of organic residuals occurs over the temperature range of $300\,^{\circ}\mathrm{C} - 350\,^{\circ}\mathrm{C}$. In the current work, the samples are baked at $500\,^{\circ}\mathrm{C}$ to burn out the organic groups. At this temperature, the structure of the sample is amorphous, and most of the organic groups can easily be removed. This procedure will be helpful in eliminating residual carbon in the coating. Without this treatment, some organics could be incorporated in the final crystal lattice. It was found that the carbon disappeared at much lower temperatures than those samples treated in a rapid sintering process since most organic groups are not burned out at low temperatures. Therefore, a higher temperature is needed to remove them. However, the

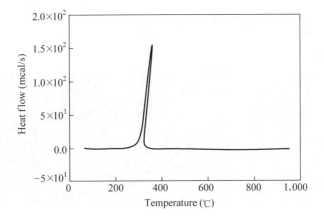

Figure 4.11 DTA profile of the HA-coating sample showing a reaction near $300\,^{\circ}\mathrm{C}$

reactivity of HA may be considerably reduced. It should be noted that the removal of the organic residue is not only related to the microstructure, but also to the macrostate of the samples. We have found that, for a thick and dense coating, high temperature will be needed in order to remove the residual carbon.

Figure 4.12 is the scanning electron microscope(SEM) micrographs showing the surfaces of the HA coating on dense alumina. As can be seen in this figure, the coating is fairly porous which will contribute to bioactivity when immersed in SBF. Figure 4.13 is SEM image of HA-coated reticulated alumina with significant open pores in the matrix. Figure 4.13(b) is the X-ray map recorded with Ca k_α lines for coated porous alumina. As can be seen in Fig. 4.13(b), the distribution of calcium demonstrated that HA is uniformly coated on the skeleton of the substrate. Figure 4.14 is the SEM micrograph showing the interface between the HA coating and the substrate. We have determined that the coating thickness was around 1 μm, which can also be altered by a second or third coating.

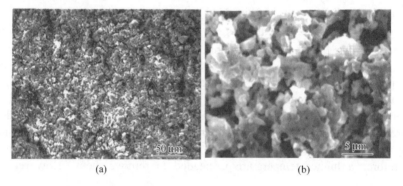

(a)   (b)

Figure 4.12 SEM photographs showing the coated HA surface on a dense alumina substrate. (a) low magnification, and (b) high magnification

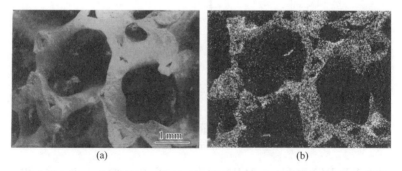

(a)   (b)

Figure 4.13 SEM photographs showing (a) porous alumina substrate and (b) an X-ray map recorded with Ca k_α lines (k_α is the characteristic spectrum of the element.)

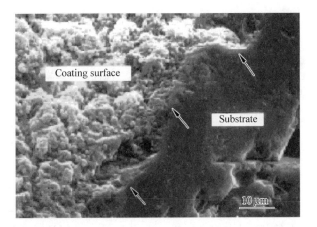

Figure 4.14 SEM photograph showing the interface between the HA coating and the dense alumina substrate

4.1.4 Coating of Hydroxyapatite Using Sol-Gel Synthesis

As a result of great advantages in sol-gel coating, despite the success in using thermal deposition (TD) method, sol-gel method was used for HA coating, and the result was proved positive. Since all bioactivity test was performed on TD samples and the coating results of sol-gel was quite similar to those of TD, only some typical results of sol-gel were shown here. Nonetheless, the importance and viability of this method need to be noted in coating HA on alumina and other ceramic substrates.

In the coating of HA, the flowchart of the sol-gel synthesis is shown in Fig. 4.15.

The hydrolysis consists of the following reaction:

$$C_6H_5-PCl_2 + H_2O \longrightarrow C_6H_5-P(OH)_2 + 2HCl$$

The polymerization process is described as:

$$C_6H_5 - P(OH)_2 \xrightarrow[-H_2O]{+O_2} -\underset{\underset{O}{\parallel}}{\overset{\overset{C_6H_5}{|}}{P}}-O-\underset{\underset{C_6H_5}{|}}{\overset{\overset{O}{\parallel}}{P}}-O-\underset{\underset{O}{\parallel}}{\overset{\overset{C_6H_5}{|}}{P}}-O-\underset{\underset{C_6H_5}{|}}{\overset{\overset{O}{\parallel}}{P}}-O-$$

The final step involves the oxidation:

$$6PO_2C_6H_5 \cdot 10CaO \xrightarrow[-\text{organic}]{+O_2} Ca_{10}(PO_4)_6(OH)_2$$

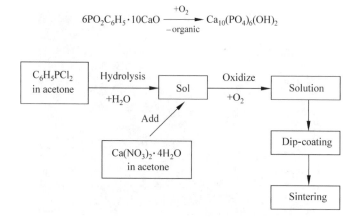

Figure 4.15 Flowchart of sol-gel synthesis for coating of HA on alumina

Following these processes, the sol-gel solution was made and coated using the procedure described in Chapter 3. The coated substrate was subsequently heat-treated to obtain a uniform HA coating on the inner pore surfaces. The microstructure of sol-gel synthesized HA coating is shown in Fig. 4.16 that is quite similar to those prepared by TD.

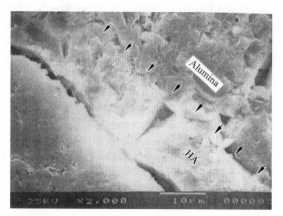

Figure 4.16 SEM photograph showing the HA coating prepared by sol-gel

4.2   Adhesion of Hydroxyapatite Film on Alumina Substrate

The bond strength between the HA coating and the substrate was determined using the tape test (ASTM D 3359), which is originally designed for organic coatings on metallic substrates. We have used this method to find out a relative bond strength. All the tests were performed on dense alumina substrates with one or multi-layer HA coating. Permacel 670 tape (Permacel, NJ, USA) was used in the test. After removal from the coating, the tape was examined under a light microscope. No peeling of the coating film was observed for all samples indicating a strong bonding between the HA coating and the substrate.

It should be noted, in testing of the adhesion strength, that we have tried to coat another type of material on alumina and carried out the tape test. This experiment was performed to investigate the adhesion behavior and to compare the tape test results. We have attempted to coat silver on the same alumina substrate using an electroless plating method.

Table 4.1 shows the tape test results on the relationship between the numbers of silver particles left on the tapes versus sintering temperature. The number of particles on the tape (NPT) after the test is normalized to 100 of the unsintered sample. A great portion of the silver film on the unsintered sample is removed by the testing tape as shown in Table 4.1. However, by sintering the sample at 400°C, NPT has dropped more than 70 percent indicating a significantly increased bonding strength due to sintering. When the sample was sintered to above 600°C, silver particles were hardly found on the tape. From these results, we conclude that sintering could significantly improve the bond strength, especially at higher temperatures. For well-sintered HA, the tape test results are similar to those of silver coating at 700°C indicating a strong bonding.

Table 4.1   Values of NPT versus sintering temperature for silver coating

NPT	Sintering Temperature (°C)	NPT	Sintering Temperature (°C)
100	20	15	500
95	200	6	600
72	300	4	700
29	400		

4.3   References

1. de Groot, K., Hydroxyapatite coating for implant in surgery. In: P. Vincezini, ed. High Tech Ceramics, Elsevier, Amsterdam, p. 381, (1987)
2. Van Raemdonk, W, P. Ducheyne. J. Am. Ceram. Soc. **6**: 381 (1984)
3. Pilliar, R., H. Cameron. BioMed. Eng. **10**: 126 (1975)
4. Maruno, S., K. Hayashi, Y. Endosseous. Dental implants of bioactive composite

materials of hydroxylapatite containing glass-coated titanium. In: T. Yamamuro and L. L. Hench, eds. Handbook of Bioactive Ceramics, Vol. 2, CRC Press, Boca Raton, FL. pp. 187 – 193(1990)
5. Holmes, R., V. Mooney, R. A. Bucholz. Clin. Orthop. **188**: 252(1984)

4.4 Problems

1. What are the essentials when involving ceramic coating on a substrate for the following requirements?
   a) The coated film needs to be uniform in thickness but without grain orientation;
   b) The coated film needs to be strongly bonded to the substrate;
   c) The coating must not be chemically reactive with the substrate.
2. List all the major ceramic thin film deposition methods including those used in semiconductor industry.
3. What would be an accurate but viable way of determining the film bonding strength to the substrate?
4. Why is the solution method used in coating the porous ceramic substrate in this chapter?
5. What is sol-gel method? Find related literature on sol-gel synthesis. Can you find other applications of sol-gel in industry and research?

5 Properties and Characterization of Biomaterials[*]

5.1 Characterization of Ceramics

Because bioceramics are used within the body, control of their composition, surface properties and microstructure is especially critical. Characterization of a biomaterial prior to exposure to *in vitro* and *in vivo* environments is also essential. The routinely used methods, i.e. X-ray diffraction (XRD), infrared spectroscopy (IR) and chemical analysis can provide valuable information on these properties. XRD determines the purity, crystallinity of the HA phase, approximate ratios of the other phases, and the lattice parameters of the HA and other phases. IR gives information to support XRD data detects additional phases, indicates relative crystallinities, and provides evidence of substituents (e. g. CO_3, F). X-ray fluorescence is suitable for the compositional analysis.

The property of vital concern for the final product is its bioactivity; i.e. ability to bond to tissues. This is a surface chemical property. There are two approaches for analyzing the mechanisms and reactions at an implant surface. First, the constituents released into a test environment or surrounding tissues can be analyzed. The traditional wet chemical methods, such as atomic emission or absorption spectroscopy, or inductively coupled plasma (ICP) chemical analysis can be applied. Solution analysis, however, provides no understanding of the changes occurring on the surface of the implant.

A second approach, surface analysis of the material, is also required to determine compositional gradients or phase changes taking place. The following summarizes the range of instrumental methods available for surface characterization.

Infrared microscopy — This is a method with high resolution and sensitivity. It can be used for the analysis of samples before and after *in vitro* or *in vivo* testing. This method gives quantitative information of the chemical composition of the surface since it is sensitive to the vibrational modes that are characteristic for each molecular constituent of the material.

Scanning electron microscopy (SEM) with energy dispersive spectrum

---

[*] Authors are Donglu Shi and Gengwei Jiang.

(EDS) — SEM with EDS is a rapid characterization method for surfaces and interfaces and is probably the most widely used instrument for this purpose. It must be noted that there is a deep sampling depth of several μm for this method. The important advantage of the SEM method is that microstructural and surface features can be observed and their dimensions and area fraction measured. The composition of the surface and microstructural features can be analyzed chemically with EDS.

Electron microprobe analysis (EMP) — This electron beam method is excellent for determining the thickness and compositional gradient of reaction layers formed on bioceramic implants. The intensity of the X-ray signal for each element (which is proportional to composition) can be obtained as a function of distance across the interface.

Auger electron spectroscopy (AES) — AES examines the outermost surface of a material with a resolution on the scale of 0.1 nm. AES combined with Ar ion milling, which removes 1 to 50 μm slices of a surface between AES analyses, is one of the most accurate methods for determining compositional gradients within the outermost layers of a bioceramic.

Surface charge analysis — The surface charge of a bioceramic influences the adsorption of proteins and other biological constituents and affects the response of tissues in contact with it. The sign and magnitude of surface charge are determined by the composition of the material, the crystal phases in the material, the defects in crystalline phases, and the pH of the solution in contact with the material. One of the most useful methods for determining surface charges of bioceramics is a zeta potential measurement. Ducheyne and coworkers discuss this method and its use in characterizing the behavior of various calcium phosphate ceramics. They have shown that the cationic defect structure of stoichiometric and Ca-deficient HA has a large effect on surface charge of the materials. The magnitude and duration of the changes in zeta potential of the apatites are related to an ion exchange between the hydrated layer around the ceramic surface and a net precipitation of new material. The zeta potential method should be considered as a characterization method for HA ceramics to determine the relative effect of defect structures on surface properties.

5.2 Bioactive Properties and Hard Tissue Prosthetics

5.2.1 Bone Biology

Bones can be categorized as short, flat, and tubular. The function of the bone is to mainly withstand the forces imposed by normal activities. Marrow, consisting of a resource of bone cells and the blood vessels, is a central fatty surrounded by bone tissue and periosteum. In the study of the bone structure, it is found that two forms of bone tissue make up the major part of the bone: cortical bone and cancellous bone [1 – 7]. These structures are differentiated by their density and mechanical strength. Cortical bone exhibits a porosity of approximately 10% while the cancellous bone possesses a much more porous structure with 50% – 90% porosity. Thus the former is significantly stronger with a compressive strength ten times higher than those of cancellous bone. Due to their porosity distributions, the mechanical behavior may differ from various types of bone. The dense cortical bone can withstand high bending stress and torsion while thinner cortices can provide greater flexibility and deformation, which are supported by cancellous bone. Therefore, the subchondral bone is able to not only form an articular surface, but also to absorb energy from sudden impact applied across the synovial joints.

For normal functionalities in mature bones, a vascular system must be able to supply the cells of the marrow, bone tissue, and periosteum. Necrosis and impair healing will occur if there is any disruption of the blood supply due to disease and injury. Therefore, in hard tissue prosthetics, the bone substitute materials must contain necessary porosity for an organization of vascular canals, which can ensure the blood supply. Furthermore, the vascular connections between the muscle and the periosteum is also important as disruption of it can cause complications during the formation of new bone.

5.2.2   Critical Issues on Interfaces Between the Hard Tissue and Biomaterials

The major effort on bioactivity studies has been on: (1) identifying the principal mechanisms that operate the interface bio-and chemical-reactions between the implant materials and soft/hard tissues, (2) studying the factors such as composition, porosity size and morphology that dominate bioreactions including bioresorbability, reaction kinetics, and ingrowth rates, and (3) mechanical properties. The concept of bioactivity was established based on the fact that an adherent layer must form between the tissue and the implant, and the bonding should possess considerable mechanical strength. It was found that several types of glasses and ceramics could directly bond to bone, but the bioactivity was found only within certain compositional limitations. The surface reaction kinetics have been found to relate to the following factors [6]: (1) surface area which is expressed in weight dissolved per unit surface area exposed, (2) porosity (usually range from 5 – 100 mm), and (3) composition of the implant. It was found that dense HA and TCP had a low tendency to bioresorb as a result of small surface area. Therefore, to induce high bioactivity, large surface area and high porosity are necessary. For effective bone ingrowth, a high porosity level of 70% is required.

5.2.3 Factors that Influence Bioreactivity

Many factors can affect bioreactivity such as composition, morphology, and porosity level. An important factor influencing bioreactivity is the surface area as it directly determines the dissolution rates of any solid materials. Currently, investigated materials are mostly porous in nature with interconnecting micro-probes in the range of from 100 to 400 μm. The porosity level is an important factor in two different biologic reactions: solution-mediated and cell-mediated processes. The former is through the implant dissolution in physiologic solutions and the latter is based on phagocytosis. It has been proposed that porosity promotes bioresorption by separating secondary to solution-mediated process. Thus, the cell-mediated process is enhanced as the partially dissolved materials are removed from the small crystals. Therefore, the denser materials tend to have lower bioresorbability due to their smaller surface area. Furthermore, the materials that have slower dissolution rates would also have lower bioresorbability such as HA. In contrast, TCP, with a high dissolution rate, has been shown to be most bioresorbable.

5.2.4 Bone Implant

Although joint replacement surgery has been very effective in the treatment of arthritic conditions, the method of attaching the prosthesis to the bone is still being developed. In implant fixation, polymers such as polymethylmethacrylate have traditionally been used. However, long term failure of fixation by using these materials has been a major concern. Therefore, noncemented techniques have been developed [8 – 17]. As an alternative, hydroxyapatite(HA) has been used for implant fixation when it is applied to the surface of a metal substrate. This has clinically been proven to be effective in short term follow-up. Despite the advantages of HA such as long term stability, HA particulates shed from the implant were observed at the implant bone interface in the autopsy studies. Particulate debris at the bone prosthesis interface results in foreign body response which is detrimental to the surrounding bone leading to implant loosening. Shedding cab be improved by optimizing the HA material properties. The high-quality HA implant fixation may prevent an aggressive osteolytic response. Another concern with HA coated implants is the strength of attachment of the HA to the metal substrate. Improved fixation strength of the HA to the metal can be achieved by employing various processing routs, coating methods, and optimizing HA synthesis. The materials approach can effectively prevent loss of fixation of the prosthesis at the metal HA interface.

5.2.5 Bonding Mechanisms

The common characteristics of bioactive materials are the formation of a Ca-P-rich layer at the interface between the implant and bone [1,2]. As reported by Kotani *et al.*, precipitation of apatite crystals is observed in Bioglass, KGS, and A-W GC [19]. They have found that there is an intervening apatite layer formed as a result of dissolution of certain components from the glassy phase present at the interface area. The layer is also observed to be collagen free with apatite crystals distinctly different from bone in terms of morphology and orientation. A Si-rich layer has also been found to exist at the interface for Bioglass and KGS, however, not observed in A-W GC and HA. Such a layer has been reported to have less mechanical strength. HA has been found to have much lower solubility compared to other biomaterials [20]. Both glassy phase and Si ions are also found to be absent at the interfaces. In a study conducted by Jarcho *et al.*, they have found that TCP dissolved in buffered acid (pH 5.2; 0.4 mol/L lactate) more than ten times faster than HA. Thus, in the TCP-HA ceramics, large proportion of TCP will result in a higher degree of bioresorbability. The formation mechanism of apatite layer for HA is belived to be different from that of Bioglass, KGS, and A-W GC. Although the morphology of the intervening layer in HA is similar to those of Bioglass, KGS, and A-W GC, its thickness is much thinner, which is consistent with its low solubility. Since TCP is considered a bioresorbable material, the bonding to bone is in direct contact without any intervening layer. From these observations, it may be concluded that the interface reaction is directly determined by the solubility, and the interface layer formation mechanisms differ drastically from various types of materials.

The property of vital concern for the final product is its bioactivity; i.e. ability to bond to tissues. This is a surface chemical property. There are two approaches for analyzing the mechanisms and reactions at an implant surface. First, the constituents released into a test environment or surrounding tissues can be analyzed. The traditional wet chemical methods, such as atomic emission or absorption spectroscopy, or inductively coupled plasma (ICP) chemical analysis can be applied. Solution analysis, however, provides no understanding of the changes occurring on the surface of the implant.

5.2.6 *In vitro* Behavior of Hydroxyapatite

Since any clinical use of calcium phosphate bioceramics involves contact with water, it is important to know the stability of HA in the presence of water at ambient temperatures. As Driessens showed, there are only two calcium phosphate materials that are stable at room temperature when in contact with aqueous solution, and it is the pH of the solution that determines which one is the most stable. At a pH lower than 4.2, the component $CaHPO_4 \cdot 2H_2O$ is the most stable, while at higher pH (>4.2), HA is the stable phase. Therefore, in the case of *in vitro* tests, at biological pH value, only HA can be found in contact with simulated body fluids(SBF).

It is believed that synthetic HA ceramic surfaces can be transformed to biological apatite through a set of reactions including dissolution, precipitation, and ion exchange. Following the introduction of HA to SBF, a partial dissolution of the surface is initiated causing the release of Ca^{2+}, HPO_4^{2-} and PO_4^{3-}, and increasing the supersaturation of the micro-environment with respect to the stable (HA) phase. Carbonated apatite can form using the calcium and phosphate ions released from partially dissolving ceramic HA and from the biological fluids that contain other electrolytes, such as CO_3^{2-} and Mg^{2+}. These become incorporated in the new CO_3^{-} apatite micro-crystals forming on the surfaces of ceramic HA crystals. The *in vitro* reactivity of HA is governed by a number of factors, which can be considered from two aspects: *in vitro* environment and properties of HA material. It is worth noting that most scientific publications deal with the former one. Intensive investigation had been done on the factors such as the type and concentration of the buffered or unbuffered solutions, pH of the solution, degree of saturation of the solution, etc. Less *in vitro* tests deal with HA material itself. Of those having been investigated, the following are the most relevant:

Defect Structure — Daculsi *et al.* reported the presence of hexagonal parallelapiped (void type) lattice defects in addition to other defect structure in crystals of ceramic HA sintered at 950°C but not in those prepared at 1,250°C [21–23]. It may be logical to assume that the differences in the amount and types of lattice defects could cause difference in reactivity *in vivo*; this assumption is in good agreement with the experimental observations reported by Niwa *et al.* that materials sintered at lower temperatures were more reactive than those sintered at higher temperature. However, no further systematic study has been done on this subject [24].

Substituted Apatite — Substitutions involved ions of F^- for OH^-, carbonate for phosphate, and Mg^{2+} or Na^+ for Ca^{2+} are of the most interest, since these substitutions are related to the biological mineralization and the development of substituted HA as new biomaterials. Substitutions result in changes in properties: e. g. lattice parameters, morphology, and solubility. Elliott and Young showed that Cl substitution causes the loss of hexagonal symmetry and exhibits monoclinic symmetry. However, this brings no change in its crystallinity. Substitution of F for OH is usually associated with an increase in the crystallinity, reflecting increase in crystal size, and imparts greater stability to the structure. This increased stability can explain why F-substituted apatites are less soluble than F-free apatites. Magnesium and carbonate have been shown to cause a decrease in crystallinity and an increase in the extent of dissolution of synthetic apatites.

Biphasic Calcium Phosphate BCP — In studies on BCP materials consisting of different β-TCP: HA ratios, it was observed that the abundance of the CO_3^- apatite microcrystals on the surfaces of the large BCP crystals was influenced by the β-TCP: HA ratio: the higher the ratio, the greater the abundance of the CO_3^- apatite micro-crystals. This was thought to be due to the higher dissolution properties of the β-TCP component of the BCP causing an increase in the concentration of the calcium and phosphate ions in the micro-environment leading to precipitation of the carbonated apatite.

The HA-coated dense alumina has been used in animal *in vivo* test. Figure 5.1 shows the interface between a HA-coated alumina and dog tubua bone. As can be seen in this figure, the interface is quite coherent without the infected area. A bone ingrowth layer has been induced at the interface indicating the superb bio-absorption of the HA coating.

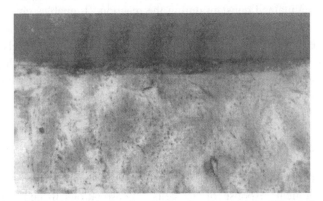

Figure 5.1 A SEM micrograph showing the interface between the HA coating and bone

5.3 Measurements of Growth and Dissolution of Hydroxyapatite Ceramics

The precipitation and dissolution of HA play an important role in the formation of biological apatite. In order to investigate the reaction mechanisms, it is important to study the growth or dissolution rates at different driving forces. Generally, there are three categories of methods developed to determine the reaction rates.

(1) Free Drift Method — This is one of the earliest experimental approaches, in which the rate of reactions obtained by following concentration changes as a function of time. The concentrations may be recorded by continuous monitoring methods or by sampling the solution suspension, filtering rapidly and analyzing for lattice ions using accepted analytical techniques.

(2) Potentiostatic Method — For some systems, it is necessary and convenient to investigate the rate of reaction when the activity of one or more species is held at a constant value. For calcium phosphate, the nature of the phases precipitating and rates of reaction are dependent upon solution pH at a given supersaturation. It is therefore an advantage to investigate these systems at constant pH using traditional pH stat procedures. The pH is maintained constant by adding acidic or basic titrant solutions controlled by a potentiostat incorporating glass and reference electrodes. The reaction rate can be evaluated from the volume of titrant consumption with time.

(3) Constant Composition Method — This is more desirable than the above two methods. In this method, the activities of all the species in the solution can be maintained constant during the reaction. It enables changes in reactivity of the crystal surfaces to be investigated as a function of time at a given driving force, and the reaction rates to be determined more precisely. Constant composition experiments involve the simultaneous addition of multiple titrants of precisely monitored volumes. Although this may be achieved with separately driven burets, it is usually preferable for them to be mechanically coupled.

5.4 *In vitro* Test Conducted in This Reasearch

In vitro tests that use cell cultures have commonly been performed to investigate the biological response of the cells. Investigations in cell-free solutions with ionic concentrations that are similar to body fluid allow the study of the chemical and mineralogical changes of the implant under conditions that simulate the physiological interactions between the material surface and the implant site. Immersion of bioactive ceramics in simulated body fluids (SBF) will result in dissolution and precipitation processes due to structural and biochemical instability of the material. Therefore, studies in simulated physiological solutions are of great importance in determining the response mechanism of the biomaterials. The objective is to investigate the chemical and morphological changes that result from immersion of HA coatings in SBF.

The *in vitro* tests were conducted to evaluate the bioactivity of the synthetic HA. All the samples were tested in powder form (Table 5.1). Two groups of samples were tested. The first one is the commercial hydroxylapatite (HA). The commercial HA samples were heat treated at 600°C (HA600) and 900°C (HA900) for 30 min, respectively. The second group of samples was prepared by a so-called thermal deposition method [25, 26]. These samples were heat treated at elevated temperatures and denoted as SHA (synthetic hydroxylapatite) 700 (heat-treated at 700°C for 4 h), SHA800 (heat-treated at 800°C for 4 h), and SHA900 (heat-treated at 900°C for 4 h). By heat-treating these samples, varied structural crystallinity was obtained in the materials.

Table 5.1 Specimen used in the *in vitro* test

Name	Source and Treatment	SSA (m^2/g)
HA	Commercial	63.02
HA600	HA heated at 600°C, 30 min	40.92
HA900	HA heated at 900°C, 30 min	17.45
SHA700	Synthesized HA heated at 700°C, 4 h	15.19
SHA800	Synthesized HA heated at 800°C, 4 h	1.49
SHA900	Synthesized HA heated at 900°C, 4 h	1.23
#1	HA heated at 700°C, 3.5 h, Particle size: 40 – 100 mesh	24.38
#2	HA heated at 700°C, 3.5 h, Particle size: 100 – 200 mesh	25.70
#3	HA heated at 700°C, 3.5 h, Particle size: < 200 mesh	27.02

An simulated body fluids (SBF) solution that had ionic concentrations close to human blood plasma, as shown in Table 5.2, was prepared by dissolving reagent-grade NaCl, $NaHCO_3$, KCl, $K_2HPO_4(3H_2O)$, $MgCl_2(3H_2O)$, $CaCl_2$, and Na_2SO_4 in ion-exchanged distilled water. The solution was buffered at pH 7.4 with 1 mol/L HCl and tris(hydroxymethyl) aminomethane $((CH_2OH)_3CNH_2)$ at 37°C. Sample powders were immersed into solution at

1×10^{-3} g/L ratio and maintained at $37°C$ at periods of time ranging from 15 min to 9 weeks. The calcium concentrations in the solutions were measured by inductively coupled plasma. Subsequent to immersion, the solutions were vacuum filtered. The powders were gently rinsed with alcohol, ion-exchanged distilled water and then dried at room temperature.

　　The surface microstructures before and after immersed in SBF solution were analyzed *via* scanning electron microscopy (SEM) (Model Hitachi, Tokyo, Japan). X-ray diffraction (XRD) and Fourier transform infrared spectroscopy (FTIR) determined the contents of the phases that were present in the coatings. Measurements were obtained on a Philips X-ray diffractometer with CuK-radiation at 35 kV and 23 mA.

Table 5.2　Ionic concentration of SBF in comparison with those of human blood plasma

	Concentration (mmol/L)							
	Na^+	K^+	Ca^{2+}	Mg^{2+}	HCO_3^-	Cl^-	HPO_4^{2-}	SO_4^{2-}
Blood plasma	142.0	5.0	2.5	1.5	27.0	103.0	1.0	0.5
SBF	142.0	5.0	2.5	1.5	4.2	147.8	1.0	0.5

5.5　Mechanical Properties

The weak mechanical properties of biomaterials have been the primary obsticles to the applications in hard tissue prosthetics. It has been reported that the strength of the porous bioactive materials is comparable to the cancellous bone [27 − 30]. For example, the compressive strength of cancellous bone and porous calcium phosphates is on the same order of 40 MPa while that of the cortical bone can reach 140 MPa [31]. The tensile strengths of cancellous bone and porous calcium phosphates are much lower, which are of the order of 5 MPa [31]. As a result of poor mechanical strength, biomaterials are precluded from common prosthetic devices such as screws, bone plates, and IM rods. The main application has been the construction of bone graft substitutes such as homograft and autograft. Other applications included extenders, which can serve as a scaffold for repair, and void filler, which is commonly used in hard tissue prosthetics. Dense bioceramics may have significantly improved mechanical properties. However, they suffer from having much lower bioreactivity due to smaller surface area. Nonetheless, the usefulness of dense ceramics is recognized particularly in maintaining surrounding bone in atrophic areas such as the edentulous alveolar ridge.

To improve the mechanical strength, various methods have been developed such as glass-ceramics composite toughened by zirconia [32] and reinforced by SiC whiskers [33]. The former employs three different zirconia powders (containing various percent of Y_2O_3 and Al_2O_3) mixed with a glass of CaO 47.7, SiO_2 43.8, P_2O_5 6.5, MgO 1.5, and CaF_2 0.5 in weight percent. The sintered composites showed significantly improved properties with doubled fracture strength σ_f. For instance, the original fracture strength σ_f of the glass-ceramic is 250 MPa, but one of the composites has a σ_f of 488 MPa. Fracture toughness K_{IC} values are also increased from 1.66 to 2.7 MPam$^{0.5}$. The improvement of mechanical properties was shown to be even more significant in composites reinforced by SiC. A composition of 50 CaO 16, P_2O_5, and SiO_2 34(wt%) was mixed with SiC whiskers and sintered at 1,000°C. The following data in Table 5.3 are used for comparison.

Table 5.3 Mechanical properties of various biomaterials and human bones

Materials	σ_f(MPa)	K_{IC}(MPam$^{0.5}$)
Glass reinforced by SiC	460	4.3
Bioglass	85	0.5
A-W GC	180	2.0
Sintered Al_2O_3	250 – 550	3.0 – 5.0
Dense HA	140	1.0
Porous HA	2.5	–
Cortical bone	100 – 190	2.2 – 4.6
Cancellous bone	41	–

As can be seen in Table 5.3, the fracture strength and fracture toughness of the SiC reinforced glass-ceramic are even higher than those of the sintered alumina. However, all these strengthened materials are dense with low, or zero porosity, which may not be desirable in many prosthetic applications. As indicated, low porosity will lead to much slower dissolution rates, and in turn adversely affect the bioresorbability and reactivity. Only when a large amount of pores are introduced into the materials, that reaction kinetics and inter-growth processes can be enhanced.

5.6 References

1. Buckwalter, J. A., R. R. Cooper. Bone structure and function. The American Academy of Orthopaedic Surgeons. **36**: 27 (1987)

5.6 References

2. Currey, J. D., The Mechanical Adeptations of Bones. Princeton. New Jercey. Princeton Unversity Press (1984)
3. Martin, R. B., D. B. Burr. Structure, Function and Adaptation of Compact Bone. New York, Raven Press (1989)
4. Recker, R. R., *Embryology, anatomy, and microstructure of bone*. In: F. L. Coe and M. J. Favus, eds. *Disorders of bone and mineral metabolism*. New York, Raven Press (1992)
5. Revell, P. A., *Pathology of Bone*. New York, Springer, p. 1 (1986)
6. Sillence, D. O., A. Senn, D. M. Danks. Genetic heterogenity in osteogenesis imperfecta. *J. Med. Genet.* **16**: 101(1979)
7. Martin, R. B., D. B. Burr. *Structure, Function and Adaptation of Compact Bone*. New York, Raven Press (1989)
8. Recker, R. R., *Embryology, anatomy, and microstructure of bone*. In: F. L. Coe and M. J. Favus, eds. *Disorders of Bone and Mineral Metabolism*. New York, Raven Press (1992)
9. Revell, P. A., Pathology of Bone. New York, Springer, p. 1(1986)
10. Sillence, D. O., A. Senn, D. M. Danks. Genetic heterogenity in osteogenesis imperfecta. *J. Med. Genet.* **16**: 101 (1979)
11. Buckwalter, J. A., *Musculoskeletal tissues and the musculoskeletal system*. In: S. L. Weinstein, and J. A. Buckwalter. eds. *Turek's orthopaedics: principles and their applications*. Philadelphia, J. B. Lippincott **5**: 13067(1994)
12. Sevitt, S., *Bone Repair and Fracture Healing in Man*. New York, Churchill Livingstone. p. 1(1981)
13. Glimcher, M. J., *The nature of the mineral component of bone and the mechanisms of calcification*. In: F. L. Coe and M. J. Favus, eds. *Disorders of Bone and Mineral Metabolism,* New York, Raven Press, p. 265(1992)
14. Rey, C., B. Collins, T. Goehl, I. R. Dickson, M. J. Glimcher, Calcif. *Tissue Internat.* **45**: 157 (1989)
15. Rowe, D. W., J. R. Shapiro. *Osteogenesis imperfecta.* In: L. V. Avioli and S. M. Krane. eds. *Metabolic Bone Disease and Clinically Related Disorders*. Philadelphia, W. B. Saunders, **2**. 659(1990)
16. Sillence, D., Osteogensis imperfecta, an expanding panorama of variants. *Clin. Orthop.* **159**: 11 (1981)
17. Triffitt, J. T., The organic matrix of bone tissue. In: M. R. Urist., Philadelphia, J. B. Lippincot, *Fundamental and Clinical Bone Physiology*, ed. p. 45(1980)
18. Kotani, S., T. Nakamura, T. Yamamuro. *J. Biomed. Mater.* Res. **26**: 1419 (1992)
19. Jarcho, M., L. J. Dombrowski, R. L. Salsbury, B. A. Bondley. *J. Dent. Res.* **57**: 917 (1978)
20. Daculsi, G., E. Goyenvalle, and E. Aguado. *Bioceramics.* **12**: 287 – 290 (1999)
21. Daculsi, G., N. Passuti, S. Martin, C. Deudon. *J. Biomed. Mater. Res.*. **24**: 379 – 396 (1990)
22. Daculsi, G., R. Z. LeGeros, E. Nery, and K. Lynch, *J. Biomed. Mater. Res.*, **23**: 883 – 894 (1989)
23. Niwa, S., K. Sawai, S. Takahashi, H. Tagai, M. Ono, Y. Fukuda. *Biomat.* **65**: (1980)
24. Jiang, G., S. Shi. *J. Biomed Mater Res (Appl. Biomater.)* **43**: 77(1998)

25. Jiang, G. , D. Shi. *J. Biomed Mater Res (Appl. Biomater.)* **48**: 117(1999)
26. Klawitter, J. J., S. F. Hulbert. *J. Biomed. Matter. Res.* **2**: 161 (1971)
27. Kasuga, T., K. Nakajima, T. Uno, M. Yoshida. : Vol. 1, CRC Press, Boca Raton, p. 137(1982)
28. Sakamoto, O., S. Ito. Vol. 1. CRC Press, Boca Raton, p. 155(1982)
29. Imai, K., T. Yuge, K. Kitano, T. Kawase, S. Saito. Vol. 1. CRC Press, Boca Raton, p. 167(1982)
30. Jarcho, M., *Clin. Orthop.* **157**: 259 (1981)
31. Kasuga, T., K. Nakajima, T. Uno, M. Yoshida. Vol. 1. CRC Press, Boca Raton, p. 137(1982)
32. Sakamoto, O. and S. Ito. Vol. 1. CRC Press, Boca Raton, p. 155(1982)

5.7　Problems

1. What is *in vitro*? What is *in vivo*? Define these terminologies.
2. What are the advantages of *in vitro* test? Under what condition we may conduct *in vivo* test?
3. On a related topic, look for the meanings for *in situ* and *ex situ*.
4. What are the basic physical principles of scanning electron microscopy (SEM), energy dispersive spectrum(EDS), electron microprobe analysis (EMP), and auger electron spectroscopy(AES)?
5. Why do the artificial bone materials have to be made in porous forms? What would be the disadvantages if they were made denser?
6. When a HA is implanted onto a hard tissue, what is the general bonding mechanism?
7. What is bioactivity and how do you measure bioactivity?

6 Bioactivity of Hydroxyapatite[*]

6.1 General Aspects

In order to produce highly strengthened porous bioactive materials for bone substitutes, two major deposition methods, suspension method and thermal deposition method, were employed to coat the inner and outer surfaces of a porous ceramic matrix. Hydroxyapatite (HA) has been uniformly coated onto both the inner and outer surfaces of reticulated alumina substrates. It has been found that the *in vitro* bioactivity of HA coatings was affected by the structural effect, which is a combination of crystallinity and specific surface area. The bioactivity was found to have been reduced at a higher degree of crystallinity, due to the high driving force for the formation of the new phase. The reaction rate was found to be proportional to the surface area. The suggested underling mechanism was that well crystallized HA surface required high driving force for the formation of hydroxy-carbonate apatite (HCA) phase.

6.2 *In vitro* Testing Materials and Preparation

Although *in vitro* tests that use cell cultures are performed to investigate the biological response of the cells, investigations in cell-free solutions with ionic concentrations that are similar to body fluid allow the study of the chemical and mineralogical changes of the implant under conditions that simulate the physiological interactions between the material surface and the implant site. As a result of the dissolution and precipitation processes, which occur on bioactive ceramic surfaces and have an important role in bone-bonding mechanisms, studies in simulated physiological solutions are of great interest in determining the response mechanism of the biomaterials. Therefore, the objective of this study is to determine the chemical and morphological changes that result from immersion of thermal deposition synthesis HA coatings in simulated body fluids

---

* Authors are Donglu Shi and Gengwei Jiang.

(SBF).

The *in vitro* tests were conducted to evaluate the bioactivity of the synthetic HA produced by our synthesis methods. All the samples were tested in the powder form. An SBF solution that had ionic concentrations close to human blood plasma, as shown in Table 5.2, was prepared by dissolving reagent-grade NaCl, NaHCO$_3$, KCl, K$_2$HPO$_4 \cdot$3H$_2$O, MgCl$_2 \cdot$3H$_2$O, CaCl$_2$, and Na$_2$SO$_4$ in ion-exchanged distilled water. The solution was buffered at pH 7.4 with 1 mol/L HCl and tris (hydroxymethyl) aminomethane ((CH$_2$OH)$_3$CNH$_2$) at 37°C. Powders were immersed into solution at 1×10^{-3} g/L ratio and maintained at 37°C at periods of time ranging from 15 min to 9 weeks. The calcium concentrations in the solutions were measured by inductively coupled plasma (ICP). Subsequent to immersion, the solutions were vacuum filtered. The powders were gently rinsed with alcohol, ion-exchanged distilled water and then dried at room temperature.

6.3   Characterization of Immersion Solution

The elemental-concentration changes of calcium in the SBF solution as a function of time are given in Figs. 6.1 and 6.2. Both HA and HA600 led to an immediate uptake of the Ca concentration. Initially, there was a high rate of ion uptake, suggesting a new phase growth on HA surface in supersaturated solution. After 24 h, with the depletion of supersaturation, the reaction proceeded at a lower rate of uptake. For HA900, there is an induction time of 60 min prior to a detectable decrease in Ca concentration, and the initial rate of Ca uptake is much lower than those of HA and HA600.

SHA (synthetic hydroxyapatite) 700 behaved similarly to HA and HA600. However, like HA900, the reaction rate was slow. The reaction of SHA800 and SHA900 significantly differed from all the above samples. During the first hour, an increase of Ca concentration was measured indicating that dissolution of SHA800 and SHA900 preceded the new phase formation. It was also noted that the rise in supersaturation for SHA900 was greater than that for SHA800. The ion uptake took place after this initial dissolution. Another difference between HA series and SHA series was that the latter took a longer time to reach the solid/solution equilibrium stage, suggesting a slower reaction rate than that of HA series. These results indicate that the nucleation and growth of HA crystals onto the coating surface is critically dependent on the crystal structure developed in the HA coatings.

Figure 6.3 represents the Ca concentration in the solution as a function of immersion time for samples #1, #2 and #3. All these samples are commercial

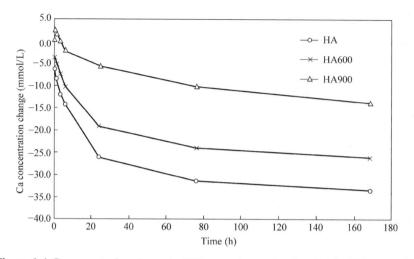

Figure 6.1 Ca concentration change in SBF versus immersion time for the HA group sintered at temperature indicated

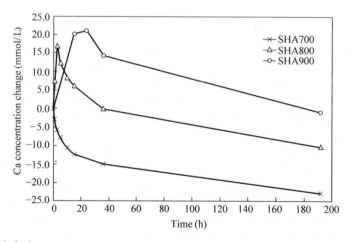

Figure 6.2 Ca concentration change in SBF versus immersion time for the synthetic hydroxyapatite(SHA) group sintered at temperature indicated

HA heat-treated at 700 °C for 30 min. Therefore, these samples are of the same structural crystallinity but with different specific surface areas. They were tested at a ratio of 1 mg/ml SBF. It is apparent in Fig. 6.3 that the rates of precipitation are highly dependent on the surface area. From these kinetic curves, the initial rate of precipitation, R_0 was determined by the slope of the first two data points. As shown in Fig. 6. 4, there is a linear relationship between the initial precipitation rate and the surface area.

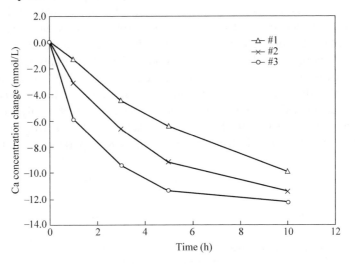

Figure 6. 3 Ca concentration change in the solution as a function of immersion time for samples #1, #2 and #3

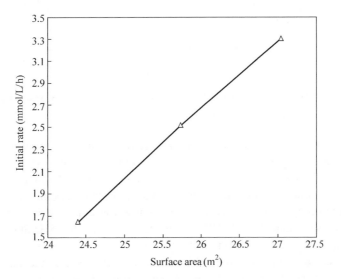

Figure 6. 4 Initial precipitation rate versus surface area for the samples showing in Fig. 6. 3

Figure 6.5 is a plot of Ca concentration verses immersion time for HA, HA600 and SHA800, SHA900. Samples of each group have been selected to have the same surface area. As can be seen, the initial rates of HA's and SHA's separate into two branches. The HA group exhibits an initial gradual decrease while that of SHA group increase quite rapidly. However, as can also be seen in this figure, calcium concentration of SHA800 initially increases, but reaches a peak at 3 h, and thereafter decreases. In SHA900, although with a different rate, the calcium concentration always increases up to 9 h. Therefore, it can be concluded that the specific surface area is not the only factor that affects the reaction behavior of various HA samples. As we will show later, the degree of crystallinity in fact plays an even more important role in the reaction rates.

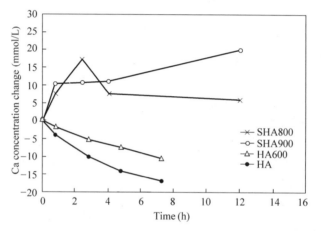

Figure 6.5 Ca concentration change versus immersion time. The first two samples have the same SA, and so do the second two

SHA700 behaves similarly to HA and HA600 with a slow reaction rate as can be seen in Fig. 6.2. However, the reaction behaviors of SHA800 and SHA900 significantly differ from the HA samples. During the first hour, an increase of Ca concentration was measured indicating that dissolution of SHA800 and SHA900 may have surpassed the new phase formation. It is noted that the rise in supersaturation for SHA900 is greater than that for SHA800. The ion uptake takes place after this initial dissolution.

Another difference between HA and SHA series is that the latter took a longer time to reach the solid/solution equilibrium stage, clearly indicating a slower reaction rate in the HA series. These results suggest that the dissolution and precipitation rates are critically dependent on the crystal structures developed in the HA samples.

6.4　Morphology of the Reacted Surfaces

Figures 6.6 and 6.7 are surfaces of SHA700 and SHA900 coatings after immersion in simulated body fluids (SBF) for 1 week and 9 weeks respectively. As can be seen, the morphology of these two surfaces is quite different. SHA700 coating was fully converted to spherulitical shapes that had a diameter of $1-10$ μm. The surface of the spherulites showed fine, needle-like structures within one week, which has been proved to be hydroxy-carbonate apatite (HCA) by infrared spectroscopy(IR) analysis. For SHA900 coating, after 9 weeks of immersion in SBF, a layer of precipitation could be observed under high magnification, which was identified as amorphous or poorly crystallized new phase instead of HCA.

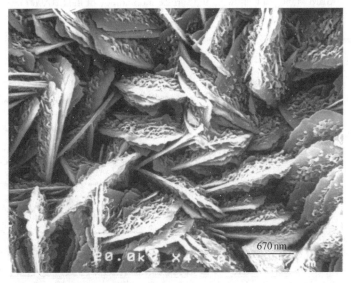

Figure 6.6 SEM photograph showing the surface morphology of the SHA700 immersed in SBF for 1 week

Figure 6.8 shows the XRD patterns of HA coatings, sintered at different temperatures in the range of 600°C to 900°C, before the immersion in SBF. The diffraction patterns have been identified for those belonging to the HA phase. Crystalline phase started to form at 600°C, and all peaks were attributed to the HA phase. Crystallite size is an indication of the crystallinity of a material

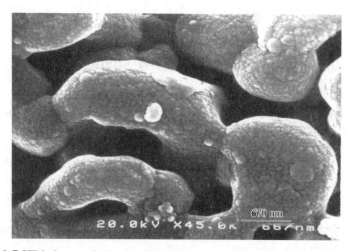

Figure 6.7 SEM photograph showing the surface morphology of the SHA900 immersed in SBF for 9 weeks

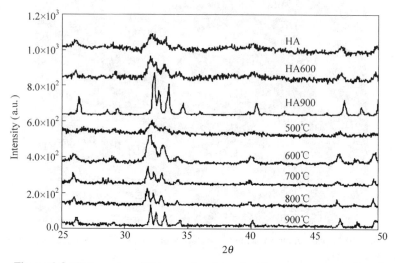

Figure 6.8 XRD spectra of HA samples sintered at the temperatures indicated

and can be defined as the average size of a domain within a material that has a coherently diffracting monocrystalline structure. The crystal size is inversely proportional to the peak width. The broadening of the peaks was evident at lower sintering temperatures, indicating the initial state of crystal formation. At higher sintering temperatures, the growth of the crystal was evidenced by the sharpening of the peaks. The peak shift could also be observed by comparing with the XRD spectra of HA900, which was considered to have been fully crystallized. At lower temperatures, in the range of 500 °C to 900 °C, the shift was significant suggesting a great lattice distortion. This structure evolution trend was also found in the samples of HA, HA600, and HA900.

Figure 6.9 shows the FTIR(Fourier transform infrared spectroscopy) spectra of an unfired sample and samples fired at 500 °C, 600 °C, 700 °C, and 900 °C. According to the standard FTIR transmission spectra [1 −3], absorption peaks observed at 3,573 and 631 cm^{-1} are assigned to monomeric OH$^-$ group stretching and vibrational modes in the apatite structure. The absorption peaks around 1,100 cm^{-1}(i.e. 1,090 cm^{-1}, 1,045 cm^{-1} and 1,040 cm^{-1} etc.) are ascribed to v_3 P—O bonds in PO_4^{3-} group in the stretching modes. The absorption peak at 960 cm^{-1} corresponds to symmetric stretching vibration of v_1 PO_4^{3-} group of hydroxyapatite and the adsorption bands around 600 cm^{-1}(i.e. 570 cm^{-1} and 605 cm^{-1} etc.) can be denoted to antisymmetric bending motion of the v_4 phosphate groups. These are characteristic peaks of HA. At a sintering temperature of 500 °C, P—O bonds formed, but hydroxyl groups were not detected. Compared with the spectra of the unfired sample, most organic groups were burned out by this temperature. At 600 °C all the characteristic lines of HA were recorded, but some organic residual could still be seen. At 700 °C and higher the peak positions match all those of standard HA, and the organic groups were not detectable.

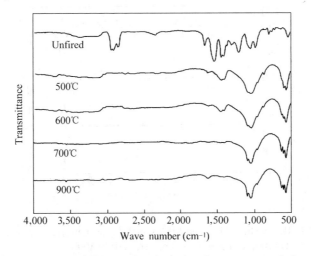

Figure 6.9 FTIR spectra of HA samples sintered at the temperature indicated for 4 h

6.4 Morphology of the Reacted Surfaces

Figure 6. 10 shows the FTIR spectra of HA and SHA powders after immersion in the SBF at time periods up to 1 week. The absorption bands at $1,460$ cm^{-1} (high C $-$ O region) and 872 cm^{-1} (low C $-$ O region) are characteristic features of hydroxy-carbonate apatite(HCA). As can be seen from the spectrum of HA (Fig. 10(c)), these bands became significantly greater after 76 h of immersion indicating an increase in carbonate content. A gradual reduction of the splitting of the major PO$_4^{3-}$ absorption bands ($1,100 - 1,000$ cm^{-1} and $600-550$ cm^{-1}) with immersion time was also observed, suggesting the formation of amorphous or fine, poorly crystallized new phases. For HA900(Fig. 6. 10(d)), a broad band appeared in the high energy C $-$ O

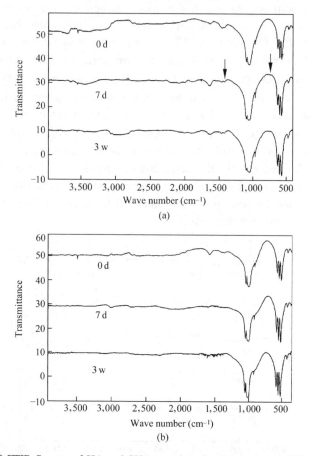

Figure 6. 10 FTIR Spectra of HA and SHA samples after immersion in SBF for the time indicated. (a) SHA700, (b) SHA900, (c) HA, (d) HA900

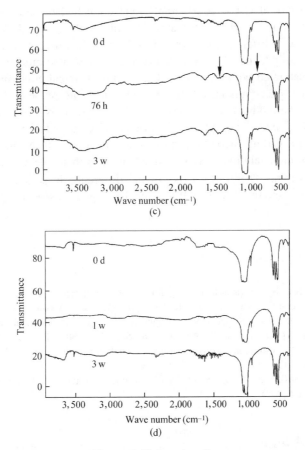

Figure 6.10 (continued)

region. However, the low energy C—O band at 872 cm^{-1} was not recorded. At the same time, a gradual reduction of the splitting of the major PO_4^{3-} bands was observed, indicating the formation of amorphous or fine, poorly crystallized new phases. HCA phase cannot be identified from these weak bands, and it is likely that some intermediate phases other than HCA have formed. HCA peaks appeared in the spectra of SHA700 within 7 days (Fig. 6.10(a)). A time-dependent increase in the carbonate band intensities accompanied by a reduction in splitting the major PO_4^{3-} bands was again recorded. Similar changes occurred in the spectra of immersed SHA800. However, no characteristic HCA peaks were recorded for SHA900 up to 3 weeks(Fig. 6.10(b)), only a broad band appeared in the high energy C—O region. This trend seems to indicate that the reactivity of HA is considerably reduced at higher temperatures.

A question arises from these experimental results: why do HA crystals, prepared through different methods, or subjected to different heat treatments behave differently? The SBF used in this work represented human plasma, and it was supersaturated with respect to HA. In this chemical environment, HA is the most stable phase among all the calcium phosphate phases, thus the HCA formation is thermodynamically possible. However, only HA, HA600, and SHA700 led to immediate uptake of Ca ions. HA900, SHA800 and SHA900 went through a partial dissolution prior to precipitation. Ducheyne [4] showed that the dissolution ability of HA is much greater than that of HA heated at 900 °C for 30 min. Therefore, it is not the difference in solubility that determined their bioactivities. We shall answer these questions in detail in the next chapter.

6.5　References

1. de Groot, K., Hydroxyapatite coating for implant in surgery. In: P. Vincezini, ed. High Tech Ceramics. Elsevier, Amsterdam, pp. 381 – 390 (1987)
2. Van Raemdonck, W., P. Ducheyne. Auger electron spectroscopic analysis of hydroxylapatite coatings on titanium. J. Am. Ceram. Soc. **6**(2): 381 – 384 (1984)
3. Pilliar, R., H. Cameron. Porous surface layered prosthetic devices. BioMed. Eng. **10**(10): 126 – 135 (1975)
4. Saggio-Woyansky, J., C. E. Scott, W. P. Minnear. American Ceramic Society Bulletin **71**: 1674 (1992)

6.6　Problems

1. Why does the HA with different synthesis history respond to SBF differently?
2. What dictates the bioactivity of HA?
3. As the HA is being heated at elevated temperatures, what has happened to its structure? If there are structural changes upon heating by what techniques you may find out these changes and how can you quantify these changes?
4. In Fig. 6.2, why does the concentration of Ca both increases in SHA800 and SHA900, but that of SHA700 decreases?
5. What kind of information can you obtain by using FTIR?

7 Hydroxyapatite Deposition Mechanisms [*]

7.1 Material Synthesis and Hydroxyapatite Coating

7.1.1 General Aspects on Chemistry, Structure, and Thermal Behavior of Hydroxyapatite

One of the primary materials employed in the film deposition on ceramic substrate is hydroxyapatite due to its superb bioactive behavior and stability. The biological applications of HA stem primarily from its composition and the nature of its structure. HA materials are composed of the same ions that make up the bulk of the natural bone mineral. Its structure belongs to the hexagonal system, with a space group, P63/m. Constructed from columns of divalent metal ions and oxygen atoms forming parallel channels in the lattice, this apatite structure is particularly prone to ion substitution to form solid solutions. As shown in Chapter 2, in HA, carbonate, CO_3 can substitute either for the hydroxyl (OH) or the phosphate (PO_4) groups, designated as Type A and Type B substitutions respectively. Type A carbonated apatite could be obtained by treating hydroxyapatite in a dry CO_2 stream, while Type B could be fabricated by precipitation from aqueous solutions. Biological apatite is referred to as Type B.

The HA powders can readily be synthesized by means of various techniques, and their characteristics vary by method. Generally speaking, there are two chemical methods: dry and wet. The dry chemical methods make use of the solid-state reactions between calcium and phosphorus compounds and have the advantage of providing stoichiometric HA powders. Wet chemical methods utilize either precipitation from mixed aqueous solutions or the hydrolysis of calcium phosphates. HA powders wet-chemically produced are generally more chemically reactive due to their high surface area and fine particle size. Nonstoichiometry and low crystallinity are also characteristics of HA obtained by

---

[*] Authors are Donglu Shi and Gengwei Jiang.

precipitation synthesis. These commercial powders exhibit glassy behavior in structure, therefore quite bioreactive. However, there has been no previous work reported on the relationship between bioactivity and structure for this compound. We have for the first time raised this issue and conducted extensive experiments on the structural effects on bioactivity of HA.

In the thermal behavior of HA, it is noteworthy that, OH^- ions remain stable in the HA structure even at high temperatures. This stability made it feasible to process HA at high temperatures.

7.1.2　Material Synthesis and Hydroxyapatite Coating

To design an implant for osteoconduction it would seem logical to mimic the architecture of the natural bone structure. An idealized bone graft substitutes would have an interconnected porous system of channels with a minimum 100 μm in diameter for bone ingrowth into ceramic structures. As shown in the introduction, to make such a structure in pure HA, its mechanical strength would be too low to have any applications, particularly for structural bone. Therefore, uniquely in this research, this novel approach has been developed in simulating a real bone structure with similar structure, porosity, bioactivity, and strength. This has been accomplished well and presented in previous chapters, by coating a thin layer of HA onto the inner surface of reticulated alumina. In this way, the skeleton of the alumina provides the mechanical strength, the high porosity satisfies the requirement for bone ingrowth, and the finally and most importantly, the thin HA coating serves as a buffer for inducing osteactivity, a fundamental step in bone implant. Furthermore, the strength and the porosity of the HA/alumina composite can be modified by changing the pore size and pore density. This freedom in structure and mechanical property manipulation is an important advantage of this novel approach. In bone implant, the bone substitute often has modulus much higher than that of bone. As implanted, the fractured bone no longer bear stress as the load is taken by high-strength substitute alloys. With reduced load on the bone structure, bone materials tend to be quickly absorbed and cannot proceed in normal growth. Orthopedic sergeant therefore desires a structural substitute that has a comparable strength to bone structure. In this way, both bone and substitute may share the similar stress for a fast ingrowth of bone structure during healing. The mechanical properties of major alloy substitutes cannot be easily altered to suit this purpose. However, in our novel approach, the pore density and size can be easily modified through processing, making it possible to fabricate substitute of bone compatible strength.

Since the *in vivio* test is beyond the subject of this chapter, no experiment has been conducted to change the pore density and size. But it is noted here that sponge processing is a simple method in changing the overall density of the reticulated ceramics. With this unique synthesis characteristic it is to be pointed out that this advantage in fabricating a biomaterial has a wide structural and property tunability.

The flowchart of coating procedure is illustrated in Chapter 4. The slurry was prepared by suspending HA particles (~ 300 mesh) and glass frits (65 wt%) in an organic binder-solvent system. The glass frits used in this work were borosilicate glasses, containing about 75 wt% of a mixture of SiO_2, B_2O_3 and 20 wt% alkali metal oxides Na_2O. They had good adhesion to the Al_2O_3 substrate and weak reaction with HA during firing. After melting, the glass was quenched in water and ground in a ball mill into glass frits of the desired particle size (~ 325 mesh). An important property of the suspension was its viscosity. Specifically, when the porous substrate was immersed in the suspension, the suspension must be fluid enough to enter, fill, and uniformly coat the substrate skeleton.

7.1.3 Coating of Hydroxyapatite onto Inner Surfaces of Pores in Reticulated Alumina

As described in the Chapter 4, the reticulated alumina has been selected as the substrate. Although there have been many coating techniques, few is applicable to coating of inner surfaces of pores. All these coating methods have been used to coat flat and dense outer surfaces of the substrate but they cannot be used for inner surface coating. For instance, spray coating and sputtering can only deposit HA films on the substrate surface while sol-gel, in its original form, may block the pores. Therefore, in this research unique coating methods have been developed for coating inner surfaces of the pores in the reticulated alumina.

7.1.4 Hydroxyapatite-Glass Slurry Method

Although this is a straightforward method, it has taken extensive experiments to develop and modify the final procedures. Initially, a simpler format of HA-slurry was used without glass additions. HA powders were mixed with binders into a slurry and coated onto the inner surfaces of the pores. This method was tried first on flat alumina substrate and to see if the coating was strong and uniform. After sintering, however, the coating was not only non-uniform, but also weakly bonded to the substrate. The non-uniformity was associated with the wetability of the HA on a smooth alumina surface during the sinterting process. The commercial HA powders had an average diameter of $3-5$ μm. There were also spherical in shape as can be seen in Fig. 7. 1. When mixed with the binders, the course nature of the particles resulted in rather poor green density in the precursor stage, estimated to be $50\%-60\%$. Due to quite different characteristics of HA and alumina, the sinterability of HA onto the smooth surface of alumina was very poor. The sintered HA coating exhibits separated clusters and the bonding was extremely weak.

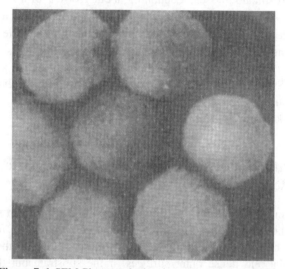

Figure 7. 1 SEM Photograph showing HA spherical particles

The poor sinterability may be understood from the point view of surface energy difference between the HA and alumina. To facilitate a sintering process, the HA particles needed to undergo the necking process in order to modify its dihedral angle, δ, as shown in Fig. 7. 2. However, as a result of the large diameter of the HA sphere, the contact area was small between the HA particle and the alumina surface. Such a small contact area had prevented the

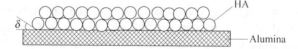

Figure 7. 2 Schematic diagram showing the sintering mechanism of large HA particles on a flat substrate

HA particles to sinter well and form a uniform layer on the alumina substrate. Two approaches in solving this problem were used.

The first one was to use a sintering aid such as a low melting point (LMP) glass. As shown in Fig. 7.3, the LMP glass would experience melting well below $1,000\,^{\circ}\mathrm{C}$ and "wet" the surface of the substrate. As the molten glass formed a cohesive interface between the HA and the alumina substrate, not only the uniformity of the HA film was improved, the bonding strength could also be increased.

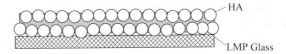

Figure 7.3 Sintering mechanism of using a LMP glass sintering aid

However, it was difficult to identify such a glass at the beginning, that would be compatible with HA and alumina. Although many types of glasses were commercially available, neither can they bone well to the substrate, nor to the HA. Therefore, a glass as sintering aid was made in the laboratory.

The glass frits used in this research were borosilicate glasses, containing about 75 wt% of a mixture of SiO_2, B_2O_3 and 20 wt% alkali metal oxides Na_2O. They had good adhesion to the Al_2O_3 substrate and weak reaction with HA during firing. The glass powders were thoroughly mixed and melted in the alumina crucible. After melting, the glass was quenched in water and ground by ball milling into glass frits of the desired particle size (~ 325 mesh). An important property of the suspension was its viscosity. Specifically, when the porous substrate was immersed in the suspension, the suspension must be fluid enough to enter, fill, and uniformly coat the substrate skeleton. This was the key in coating inner surfaces of the pores in the reticulated alumina.

The second approach was to reduce the HA particle size. It was believed that if the diameter of the HA was reduced to the order of the alumina surface roughness, that could modify the dihedral angle, and in turn enhance sinteribility. Another concern was the possible incompatibility between the glass and human hard tissue. Although HA has been well studied for its bioactivity and biocompatibility, no study has been reported on the bio-behavior of the special glass that was fabricated in the laboratory. To ensure biocompatibility, it was decided to remove all glass sintering aid from the HA coatings. For both of these reasons, it was important to seek for a better and safer way of coating a pure HA film onto the inner surfaces of the pores in reticulated alumina. But note here that the coating experiments on HA-glass slurry coating was an important step based on which this research progressed into a new stage of coating method, namely, thermal deposition (TD).

7.1.5   Thermal Deposition and Sol-Gel Methods

In general the chemical solution method has been widely used in film deposition on a variety of substrates. The common characteristics of this method is that a chemical solution either a polymeric suspension or a sol-gel solution can be made to have a low viscosity. The suspension of this nature can be used to deposit films that are not only very uniform but also with a small thickness (a few micron) depending upon the property of the substrate and the number of coating layers. Such a characteristic is perfect for coating inner surfaces of pores, particularly small pores. Another important characteristic is that the solution method deposits a film via a precipitation of the stoichiometric compound during heat treatment. The precipitate, if well controlled, can have very fine dimensions that are often needed in some specific applications. In coating the inner pore surfaces, to enhance wetability of the HA particles, much smaller particle size is preferred since the contact area between the HA and the alumina substrate is significantly increased. In the case of HA-glass slurry method, the HA particles remain their large dimensions and a strong bonding could not be achieved unless the sintering aid was employed. However, in the thermal deposition method, the strong bonding of HA has been achieved without using a sintering aid of any kind.

In the thermal decomposition (TD) method calcium 2-ethyl hexanoate was mixed with Bis(2-ethyhexyl) phosphite stoichiometrically in ethanol. The viscosity of the solution was controlled by the quantity of ethanol added. The mixture was stirred for 2 days at room temperature. The solution was used for coating both dense and porous alumina. The coated substrates were then air-dried and calcinated up to $1,000\,^{\circ}\mathrm{C}$ at a heating rate of $2\,^{\circ}\mathrm{C}/\mathrm{min}$.

To understand the enhanced wetability of HA on the alumina substrate, we may consider the surface tension associated with forming a spherical HA precipitate from the solution on a flat alumina substrate. Assuming the HA particle forms a spherical cap on the alumina subface (see Fig. 7. 4), that is, the HA is a portion of the sphere having radius r_{ab}. A top view of Fig. 7. 4 would show the HA particle as a circle with projected radius R. The question now is: what is the change in surface energy produced by the formation of the HA particle on the surface of aluminia? Taking the surface free energy equal to the surface tension and we have [1], Eq. (7. 1)

$$\Delta G = (A_{\alpha\beta}\gamma_{\alpha\beta} + A_{\beta\omega}\gamma_{\beta\omega}) - A_{\beta\omega}\gamma_{\alpha\omega} \qquad (7.1)$$

where $A_{\alpha\omega}$ is the area of the α-β interface, $A_{\beta\omega}$ is the area of the β-ω interface, and γ is the surface tension. Here β is HA and ω is alumina. Notice that the surface energy of the α-ω interface that was wiped out when the HA phase was formed, and the area of this wiped-out α-ω interface is exactly $A_{\beta\omega}$. To proceed, we construct the "surface tension force balance" at the three phases shown in Fig. 7.5.

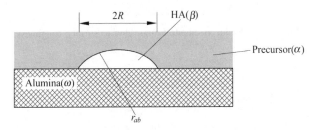

Figure 7.4 Schematic diagram showing the geometry of the spherical cap

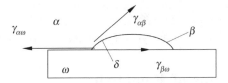

Figure 7.5 Surface tension diagram at the edge of the cap

In coating HA, one desires the HA particle to wet the surface with minimum thermal energy. Consequently, according to the above model, one desires the HA particle to have a very small dihedral angle δ with the alumina surface. This requires a small value of $\gamma_{HA\text{-}alumina}$. It should be clear that interfaces of small γ are characterized by a fairly good crystal matching at the interface. Both HA and alumina have the hexagonal lattice structures which should contribute to the reduction in δ and γ. Therefore, it is energetically much easier for the small HA precipitates to nucleate and grow on the alumina surface and form a uniform film. Furthermore, since the substrate is a curved inner surface of a pore, whose roughness may be of the order of the precipitate size, the dihedral angle is further reduced (see Fig. 7.6). As a result, the thermal deposition(TD) method has resulted in a uniform film with strong bonding strength as indicated in the previous chapters. The film deposition process may be illustrated in Fig. 7.7.

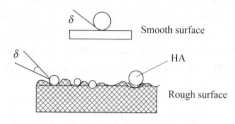

Figure 7.6 Reduced dihedral angle due to surface roughness

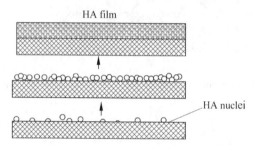

Figure 7.7 Precipitation and film growth mechanism in thermal deposition method

7.2 Mechanisms of Bioactivity

7.2.1 *In vitro* Biochemistry Behavior of Hydroxyapatite

The formation of biological apatite on the surface of implanted synthetic calcium phosphate ceramics goes through a sequence of chemical reactions. It has been shown that the reaction rate *in vitro* appears to correlate with the rate of apatite mineral formation *in vivo*. Therefore, the laboratory observations can be projected to the *in vivo* situation.

The *in vitro* behavior of bioceramics is determined by its stability at ambient and body temperatures. Many factors have significant influence on their stability, including the pH and supersaturation of the solution, crystalinity, structure defects, and porosity of the material [2, 3]. Driessens [4] showed that, among the phases composed of calcium and phosphate, hydroxyapatite (HA) is the most stable at room temperature when in contact with simulated body fluid (SBF), which was used to represent the ionic concentrations of plasma. Generally, SBF will initiate a partial dissolution of the HA material causing the release of Ca^{2+}, HPO_4^{2-} and PO_4^{3-}, and increasing the supersaturation of the micro-environment with respect to HA phase which are stable in this environment. Following this initial dissolution is the reprecipitation. Carbonate ions, together with other electrolytes, which are from the biological fluids, become incorporated in the new apatite microcrystals forming on the surfaces of the ceramic HA (Fig. 7.8).

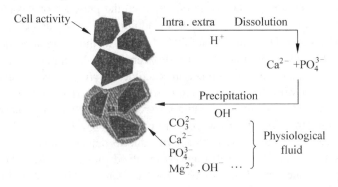

Figure 7.8 Schematic representation of the dissolution/precipitation processes involved in the *in vitro* formation of CO^{3-} apatite on surfaces of HA materials

Since any clinical use of calcium phosphate bioceramics involves contact with water, it is important to understand the stability of HA in the presence of water at ambient temperatures. As Driessens showed, there are only two calcium phosphate materials that are stable at room temperature when in contact with aqueous solution, and it is the pH of the solution that determines which one is the most stable [4]. At a pH lower than 4.2, the component $CaHPO_4 \cdot 2H_2O$ is the most stable, while at higher pH (>4.2), HA is the stable phase. Therefore, in the case of *in vitro* test, at biological pH value, only HA can be found in contact with SBF.

It is believed that synthetic HA ceramic surfaces can be transformed to biological apatite through a set of reactions including dissolution, precipitation, and ion exchange. Following the introduction of HA to SBF, an partial dissolution of the surface is initiated causing the release of Ca^{2+}, HPO_4^{2-} and PO_4^{3-}, and increasing the supersaturation of the micro-environment with respect to the stable (HA) phase. Carbonated apatite can form using the calcium and phosphate ions released from partially dissolving ceramic HA and from the biological fluids, which contain other electrolytes, such as CO_3^{2-} and Mg^{2+}. These become incorporated in the new CO_3^{2-} apatite micro-crystals forming on the surfaces of ceramic HA crystals. The *in vitro* reactivity of HA is governed by a number of factors, which can be considered from the two aspects: *in vitro* environment and properties of HA material. It is worth nothing that most scientific publications deal with the former one. Intensive investigation had been carried out on the factors such as the type and concentration of the buffered or unbuffered solutions, pH of the solution, and degree of saturation of the solution. Less *in vitro* tests deal with HA material itself. Of those having been investigated, the following are the most relevant in this study:

Defect Structure — Daculsi *et al.* reported the presence of hexagonal parallelapiped (void type) lattice defects in addition to other defect structure in crystals of ceramic HA sintered at $950°C$ but not in those prepared at $1,250°C$ [5]. It is logical to assume that the differences in the amount and types of lattice defects could cause difference in reactivity *in vivo*. This assumption is in good agreement with the experimental observations reported by Niwa *et al.* that materials sintered at lower temperatures were more reactive than those sintered at higher temperature [6]. However, no explanation was provided as to what was responsible for such varied bioactivity due to defect structures.

Substituted Apatite — Substitutions involved ions of F^- for OH^-, carbonate for phosphate, and Mg^{2+} or Na^+ for Ca^{2+} are of the most interest, since these substitutions are related to the biological mineralization and the development of substituted HA as new biomaterials. Substitutions result in changes in properties: e. g. lattice parameters, morphology, and solubility. Elliott and Young showed that Cl substitution causes the loss of hexagonal symmetry and exhibits monoclinic symmetry. However, this brings no change in its crystallinity [7]. Substitution of F for OH is usually associated with an increase in the crystallinity, reflecting increase in crystal size, and imparts greater stability to the structure. This increased stability can explain why F-substituted apatites are less soluble than F-free apatites. Magnesium and carbonate have been shown to cause a decrease in crystallinity and an increase in the extent of dissolution of synthetic apatites.

Biphasic Calcium Phosphate (BCP) — In studies on BCP materials consisting of different β-TCP/HA ratios, it was observed that the abundance of the CO_3^- apatite microcrystals on the surfaces of the large BCP crystals was influenced by the β-TCP/HA ratio. The higher the ratio, the greater the abundance of the CO_3^- apatite micro-crystals. This was thought to be due to the higher dissolution properties of the β-TCP component of the BCP causing an increase in the concentration of the calcium and phosphate ions in the micro-environment leading to the precipitation of the carbonated apatite.

7.2.2 Growth — Dissolution Mechanism

The growth and dissolution of a crystalline phase can be regarded as two opposing processes. When the HA crystal is brought into contact with a solution, its ability to grow or dissolve depends upon the value of the Gibbs free energy of the corresponding reaction. The driving force for the crystallization of the calcium phosphate phases from the solution may be expressed as Gibbs free energy, ΔG, from a supersaturated solution to a saturated one:

$$- \Delta G = (RT/\nu) \ln(IP/K_{so}) = (RT/\nu) \ln S \qquad (7.2)$$

where R is gas constant, T is temperture, IP is the ionic activity product in the supersaturated solution, K_{so} is the value of IP at equilibrium, and ν is the number of ions in the molecule. The values of IP for HA is given by Eq. (7.3)

$$IP = [Ca^{2+}]^{10}[PO_4^{3-}]^6[OH]^2 \, y_1^2 y_2^{10} y_3^6 \qquad (7.3)$$

where y_z is the activity coefficient of z-valent ionic species. The driving force for crystallization can also be expressed in terms of the degree of supersaturation, σ, given by Eq. (7.4)

$$\sigma = (IP1/\nu - K_{so}1/\nu)/K_{so}1/\nu = S - 1 \qquad (7.4)$$

where S is the supersaturation ratio. When $S > 1$, σ is positive, the solution is supersaturated and growth may occur. In contrast, when $S < 1$, the dissolution may take place in the undersaturated solution.

In solutions in which there are significant ion association and complexation, the free ion concentrations are considerably lower than the total stoichiometric values. In order to calculate S or σ using Eq. (7.3) and Eq. (7.4), it is necessary to know the concentrations of free lattice ions and their activity coefficients. The latter are functions of ionic strength, I, given by Eq. (7.5)

$$I = (1/2)(Z_j^2 C_j) \qquad (7.5)$$

where C_j and Z_j are the concentration and charge of ion species, respectively.

For most cases involving mixed electrolytes, the empirical extension of the Debye-Huckel equation proposed by Davies may be used for calculation of activity coefficients, y_j given by Eq. (7.6)

$$\lg y_j = - A_j^2 [I^{1/2}/(1 + I^{1/2}) - 0.3I] \qquad (7.6)$$

where A is a temperature dependent constant ($A = 0.5115$ at $25\,^{\circ}C$). Concentrations of the ionic species in the solutions were calculated from mass balance, electroneutrality, proton dissociation, and calcium phosphate ion-pair association constants by successive approximations for the ionic strength, I.

7.2.3 Kinetics Models for Crystallization and Dissolution

Once the nucleation has happened, the supersaturation is rapidly depleted and these crystallites will tend to grow by a process of crystal growth. The rate of crystallization can be represented in terms of the simple empirical kinetics[8]: Eq. (7.7)

$$R_g = k_g s \sigma^n \tag{7.7}$$

where k_g is the rate constant for crystal growth, s is the surface area, which is a function of the total number of available growth sites, and n is the effective order of reaction. There are nine rate-determining steps in the process of crystal growth [9]. Figure 7.9 is an illustration of each step which is described in the following:

(1) Transport of lattice ions to the surface by convection (A);

(2) Transport of lattice ions to the crystal surface by diffusion through the solution (A);

(3) Integration into the adsorption layer (B);

(4) Adsorption at the solid liquid interface (C);

(5) Diffusion within the hydrated adsorption layer (D);

(6) Adsorption at a step representing the emergence of a lattice dislocation at the crystal surface [E(I)];

(7) Migration along the step;

(8) Integration at a kink site on the step [E(II), and D];

(9) Partial or total dehydration of ions.

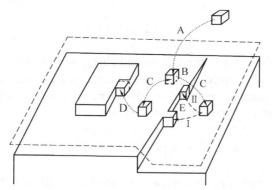

Figure 7.9 Typical crystal surface showing a dislocation, steps, kinks and absorbed growth

In each step, the following process is important in understanding the kinetics of growth and dissolution:

Mass Transport — When surface processes such as adsorption, surface diffusion, and integration and surface nucleation are extremely fast, the entire process is controlled by mass transport (steps 1 or 2 above). The growth rate will be given by Eq. (7.8):

$$V_g = k_d(S - 1).$$

$$(7.8)$$

This would lead to reaction order of unity with respect to the relative supersaturation. An expression for the rate constant, k_d, can be obtained using Fickís first law of diffusion and the classic volume diffusion model leading to Eq. (7.9):

$$k_d = DC_s/\lambda$$

$$(7.9)$$

where D is the mean diffusion coefficient of the crystalline lattice ions in solution, C_s is the solubility of the precipitating phase, and λ is the thickness of the diffusion layer at the crystal surface, which can be estimated by Eq. (7.10):

$$\lambda \sim 5.74 \, r^{0.145} (\Delta\rho)^{-0.285}$$

$$(7.10)$$

where r is the crystal radius and $\Delta\rho$ is the difference in density between solid and solution. The controlling factor can be found out by comparing the experimental rate of crystal growth with the limiting mass transport rate. If the two are of the same order of the magnitude, then it can be concluded that the crystal growth is strongly influenced by mass transport. In most cases, however, the experimental rate of crystal growth is found to be considerably less than that calculated for pure mass transport control and crystal growth is dominated by surface process involving adsorption and integration into the crystal.

Adsorption and Surface Diffusion — In Fig. 7.9, the adsorption of ions at the crystal surface may result in the formation of hydrated monolayer, which exchanges ions with the crystal lattice and the bulk solution. If the transport of growth units in the solution to the surface is so rapid that the effective concentration of the solution adjacent to this adsorbed layer is equal to the bulk value, the growth rate is controlled by processes such as adsorption, subsequent surface diffusion and integration. If a growth unit is accommodated by kink immediately after diffusing to the step, the growth rate of a surface with a screw dislocation is controlled by adsorption and surface diffusion, and the elementary growth rate (V_g) controlling process is given by Eq. (7.11):

$$V_g = k_{ad}(S - 1) \qquad (7.11)$$

where the overall reaction order is unity with respect to the relative supersaturation. The rate constant for adsorption k_{ad} has been approximated by Eq. (7.12):

$$k_{ad} = \alpha \nu_{ad} V_m C_s \qquad (7.12)$$

where α is the jump distance; ν_{ad} is the jump frequency of an ion into the adsorption layer; V_m is the molar volume of the crystalline material. The rate constant is probably also dependent upon the partial dehydration of adsorbing ions and the detailed structure of the solution/crystal interface.

Spiral Controlled Growth — A crystal fault known to exist in most crystals. In Fig. 7.9, steps may originate as dislocations or imperfections in the crystal lattice. If growth units are incorporated along the step at a uniform rate, the step winds itself into a spiral thereby providing a continuous source of growth sites on the crystal surface. At low supersaturation, the growth rate of crystal is given by an equation of the form Eq. (7.13):

$$V_g \sim k (S - 1)^2 \qquad (7.13)$$

where the effective order of reaction with respect to the relative supersaturation is 2. In simple terms, this kinetics equation can be understood as follows. The density of steps is proportional to $\ln S$ and the rate of lateral movement over the surface of the crystal is proportional to $(S - 1)$. The total rate of growth will therefore be proportional to $(S - 1)\ln S$, which, for small values of S is close to $(S - 1)^2$.

Surface Nucleation — The growth on a defect-free crystal surface is realized by the spreading of two-dimensional nuclei across the surface at moderately high supersaturations. When the crystal surface is very small, as soon as a critical nucleus forms, it may cover the entire surface before renucleation, as described by the so-called mononucleation model. However, a much more likely mechanism is that of polynucleation in which it is assumed that the crystal surface is covered by islands or surface nuclei, the edges of which form steps with kinks in which lattice ions can be readily integrated. The resulting birth and spread model leads to a rate Eq. (7.14):

$$V_g = K_p f(S) \exp(- K_p/\ln S) \qquad (7.14)$$

where the two constants are given by Eq. (7.15) and Eq. (7.16):

$$f(S) = S^{7/6}(S - 1)^{2/3}(\ln S)^{1/6} \qquad (7.15)$$
$$K_p = \pi \gamma^2 / 3(kT)^2 \qquad (7.16)$$

and K_p is the polynucleation rate constant, k is Bolzman constant, T is tempreture. The effective reaction order for polynucleation control growth is more strongly dependent upon the driving force than that for surface spiral controlled growth, and the value of order will be greater than 2.

7.2.4   Experimental Determination of Reaction Mechanisms

It is possible that the crystal growth rate is controlled by more than one of the elementary rate controlling mechanisms. The rate controlling process can change depending upon particle size, solution concentration, and surface properties of the crystallites. The mechanisms of crystal growth are usually interpreted from the measured reaction rates at different driving forces or from the activation energies of reactions.

The kinetics data can be confronted with theoretical models such as those discussed above to determine the most probable mechanism. It is common practice to fit the data to an empirical rate law, which is represented by Eq. (7.7). A broad empirical-test for growth mechanism can be achieved from a logarithmic plot of Eq. (7.7). From the n value, the probable mechanism can be deduced. It is possible that the crystal growth rate is controlled by more than one of the elementary rate controlling mechanisms listed above. Under these circumstances, the rate limiting steps may be dependent upon the jump frequency of lattice ions: (1) through the solution for mass transport control; (2) to the crystal surface for adsorption control, or (3) along the crystal surface or into a crystal lattice kink site for spiral and polynuclear control. The rate controlling process can change depending upon particle size, solution concentration, and surface properties of the crystallites. A broad empirical test for growth mechanism can be achieved by plotting the data according to Eq. (7.7). An effective order reaction in the range $0 < n < 1.2$, $n \sim 2$, or $n > 2.5$ indicates that the rate controlling process is one of adsorption and/or mass transport, surface spiral, or polynucleation, respectively. Experimentally, it is found that the growth rates of the calcium phosphates are insensitive to changes in fluid dynamics indicating surface controlling mechanisms rather than mass transport of ions to the crystal surfaces.

Activation energies, obtained from experiments at different temperatures, may be used to differentiate between volume diffusion and surface controlled processes. The activation energy for volume diffusion, reflecting the temperature dependence of the diffusion coefficient, usually lies between 16 and

20 kJ/mol, while for a surface reaction the value may be in excess of 35 kJ/mol. If a reaction has an activation energy of less than 20 kJ/mol, it is safe to assume that it is overwhelmingly controlled by volume diffusion. However, if the activation energy is higher than 35 kJ/mol, it is quite certain that an adsorption process predominates. In all other cases, both adsorption and volume diffusion mechanisms may participate for a first order reaction.

7.2.5 Effect of Heat Treatment on Hydroxyapatite

Based on the XRD spectra of HA sintered at different temperatures in the range of 600 °C to 900 °C in Fig. 4.10 of Chapter 4, we can see the structural evolution from the amorphous state during the heat treatment. The breadth of the peaks can be used as an indicator of crystal dimension in the direction perpendicular to the diffracting plane (hkl). The crystal size D is inversely proportional to the peak breadth according to the Scherer Eq. (7.17)

$$D_{hkl} = \frac{K\lambda}{\Delta(2\theta)\cos\theta} \tag{7.17}$$

where D_{hkl} is the crystallite dimension; K is the Scherer constant (here $K = 0.9$); λ is the X-ray wavelength in Angstroms; $\Delta(2\theta)$ is the true broadening of the diffraction peak at half maximum intensity. The contribution to the peak breadth from instrumental broadening was determined to be $\sim 0.12°$ (0.002 radians), independent of 2θ. This amount subtracted from the total experimental width is the value of true broadening, assuming the two contributions add linearly. The peak breadth (D002) is given as a function of temperature in Fig. 7.10. It can be seen that the peak breadth decreases with sintering temperature, indicating that the crystal size increases with increasing sintering temperature, from 600 °C to 900 °C. On the basis of the above analysis, one can see the strong effect of annealing temperature on the size and faction of the crystals.

Figure 7.11 shows the grain size of HA coatings sintered for 4 h at 700 °C, 800 °C and 900 °C, respectively. It is very obvious that the grain size increased with the sintering temperatures, and the grain size of SHA900 was twice as big as that of SHA700. Less grain boundaries can be seen from the microstructure of SHA900. Roughness of the surface was another difference among these coatings. It was likely that SHA900 coating was over-sintered, and some liquid phase might exist.

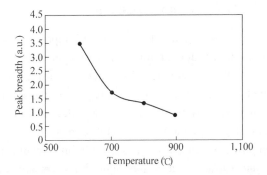

Figure 7.10 X-ray peak breadth versus temperature for the HA synthesized in this study. The solid line is a guide to eyes

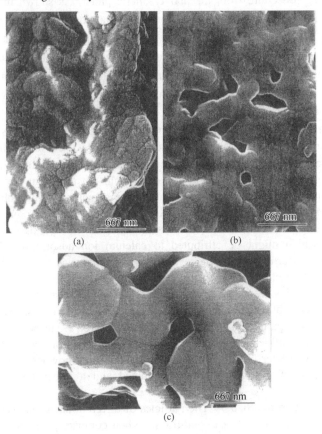

(a)   (b)

(c)

Figure 7.11 Microstructure of HA coatings sintered for 4 hrs at (a) 700°C, (b) 800°C, and (c) 900°C

7.2.6 Structural Effect on Bioactivity

Effect of Surface Area — Fig. 6.5 (in Chapter 6) represents the Ca concentration in solutions as a function of immersion time at different surface areas. These samples were the same kind of powders to ensure that they have the same crystal structure and surface morphology, while the ratio of surface area to volume of simulated body fluids (SBF) was different. It is apparent in Fig. 6.1 that the rates of precipitation were highly dependent on the surface area. Based on the empirical kinetics Eq. (7.7), to build a relationship between the reaction rate R_g and surface area s, the degree of supersaturation σ should be kept at a constant value. The corresponding reaction rates were calculated by a simple fitting procedure from the above kinetic plots. As shown in Fig. 6.4, there was a linear relationship between the precipitation rates and the total surface area, which is in agreement with the above empirical kinetics equation. This result also showed that crystallization occurred only on the added seed materials without any secondary nucleation or spontaneous precipitation. Furthermore, the advantage of porous bioceramics over dense bioceramics was proved by this relationship.

The initial precipitation rate was not used here because of the following considerations. First, the empirical fitting procedure used to calculate R_0 is greatly affected by the slower rates occurring after the initial fast stage of the precipitation process. Thus, the fitting data could not represent the true initial rate. Second, initial rate was a very complicating factor. Rapid adjustment of surface composition usually happened when the solids were introduced into the growth or dissolution media. In the case of HA, initial uptaking surges were observed, which might be attributed to calcium ion adsorption. Therefore, considerable uncertainties can arise if too much emphasis is placed upon the initial rates of reaction.

Another point needed to be noted was that in this test, the different surface areas were not originated from the distribution of particle sizes, considering that different particle sizes might bring in the factor of surface morphology, which has great influence on the reaction rate. The effect of particle size would be demonstrated later. In the current method, the same powders were used, so that the factor of morphology was eliminated and a linear relationship was obtained.

Effect of Particle Size — The particles of different sizes behaved differently under the same SA : V test conditions. When comparing the 40 – 100 mesh and <200 mesh particles at SA : V of 0.02 m^2/ml, it is apparent that the Ca adsorption rate is slower for the smaller particles. This may be attributed to the physical differences such as the radius of curvature and surface roughness.

Effect of Crystallinity — Figure 6.5 (in Chapter 6) is a plot of Ca concentration verses immersion time for HA, HA600, SHA800 and SHA900. Samples of each group were tested under the same SA:V ratio. As can be seen, the initial rate of HA was greater than that of HA600; the behavior of SHA800 differed from the one of SHA900. Therefore, it can be concluded that the specific surface area was not the only reason that affects the reaction behavior of various HA powders. The degree of crystallinity played an important role in their reaction rates.

7.2.7   Temperature Effect on Bioactivity

Figure 7.12 through Fig.7.15 show the calcium concentration change as a function of time at different temperatures for samples of HA, HA600, HA900, and SHA700. It was apparent that the reaction rates were faster at higher temperatures.

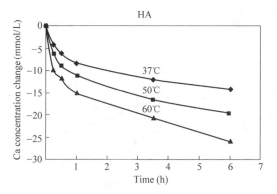

Figure 7.12 Ca concentration change versus immersion time at the temperature indicated for HA

Chemical reactions, specifically in this case, the process of nucleation and crystal growth from solution is described as an activated process with temperature, which is represented by the following relationship:

$$\text{rate} \propto \exp\left(-\frac{E_a}{kT}\right) \qquad (7.18)$$

where E_a is the activation energy, so that reaction rate increases exponentially with temperature increase. The reaction rate constant K is related to temperature

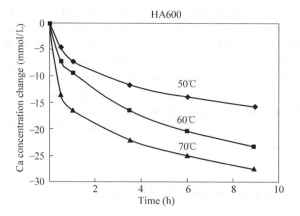

Figure 7.13 Ca concentration change versus immersion time at the temperature indicated for HA600

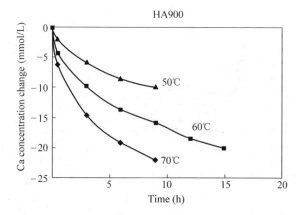

Figure 7.14 Ca concentration change versus immersion time at the temperature indicated for HA900

by an Arrhenius equation:

$$K = K_0 \exp\left(-\frac{E_a}{kT}\right) \tag{7.19}$$

Substituting Eq. (7.19) to Eq. (7.7) and taking natural logarithms of both sides, we can rewrite the Eq. (7.20) as:

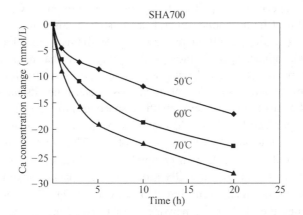

Figure 7.15 Ca concentration change versus immersion time at the temperature indicated for SHA700

$$\ln R = -\frac{E_a}{kT} + \ln(s\sigma^n) + \ln K_0 \qquad (7.20)$$

By keeping σ at a constant value, plot $\ln R$ versus $1/T$, the slope of the curve will be minus E_a/k, and consequently E_a can be calculated.

According to the procedures described above, activation energy is computed for HA, HA600, HA900 and SHA700. σ is selected at $\Delta Ca = -8$ mmol/L for all the reaction temperatures. The computed activation energy is listed in Table 7.1.

Table 7.1 Activation energies for the samples indicated

Sample	Activation Energy (kJ/mol)
HA	66.3
HA600	80.3
HA900	172.7
SHA700	130.4

The above results show that the activation energy increased with the sintering temperature for HA powders. The activation energy of synthesized HA700 is much higher than that of HA and HA600.

7.2.8 Factors Contributing to Reactivity of Hydroxyapatite

Composition and Structure — The rationale for using HA as a bone substitute material is its similarity to the inorganic component of natural bone structure.

7.2 Mechanisms of Bioactivity

Both infrared spectroscopy (IR) absorption spectrum and X-ray diffraction (XRD) pattern of human bone mineral demonstrated this similarity.

According to the definition proposed by Williams, bioactive denotes "a material which induces specific biological activity", so that bioactive materials are able to form a strong bond with host bone. The HA structure, providing chemical stability and hospitality for alien ions, determines its bioactivity. HA belongs to the hexagonal system, with a space group, $P6_3/m$. This space group is characterized by a six-fold c-axis perpendicular to three equivalent a-axes (a_1, a_2, a_3) at angles 120° to each other. The smallest building unit, known as the unit cell, contains a complete representation of the apatite crystal, consisting of Ca, PO_4, and OH groups closely packed together in an arrangement shown in Fig. 2.2 and Fig. 2.3 (in Chapter 2). The network of PO_4 groups provides the skeletal framework, which gives the apatite structure its stability. This is reflected on its solubility. Figure 7.16 shows the solubility of materials composed of calcium and phosphate in the presence of water. At pH higher than 4.2 (physiological pH), HA is the stable phase. Therefore, if there is a saturated existing with respect to the unstable phase, this solution should then be supersaturated with respect to the HA phase which makes the precipitation of new apatite thermodynamically possible. Furthermore, the HA structure allows the substitutions of many other ions, so that the biological ions, such as Mg^{2+}, CO_3^{2-}, etc. can be incorporated into the newly formed apatite, leading to the formation of biological apatite.

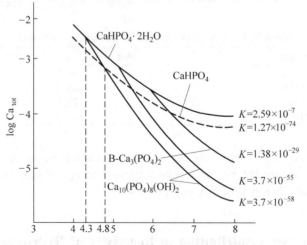

Figure 7.16 Solubility of materials composed of calcium and phosphate in the presence of water

The formation of biological hydroxy-carbonate apatite (HCA) is believed to be a dissolution-precipitation process. The role of Ca and PO_4 in HA is to aid the nucleation of the HCA phase on the surface, because body fluid will generally induce a partial dissolution of HA so that the supersaturation of the micro-environment with respect to HA is increased, promoting the precipitation of HCA phase. However, the presence of Ca and PO_4 in the implant materials may not be the critical condition for its bioactivity. Kokubo and co-workers have shown that phosphate-free glasses as well as glass-ceramics may still be bioactive [10]. The results of this research showed that same HA materials subjected to different heat treatments might present different degree of bioreactivity; some may even behave like bio-inert material. The underlying reason will be analyzed from the view of surface energy.

With respect to the role of — OH group in the bioactivity of HA, the discussion may proceed from the following aspects:

First, let's compare the bioactivity of HA with that of oxyhydroxyapatite (OHA), which was prepared by heating HA in high vacuum (10^{-7} mm(Hg)) at 900 °C for 24 h, leading to dehydroxylation. OHA can be presented by the formula:

$$Ca_{10}(PO_4)_6(OH)_2^{-2x}O_x[\ ]_x \qquad (7.21)$$

where [ ] stands for a vacancy. It can be seen as a bivalent oxygen ion and a vacancy substitute for two monovalent OH^- ions. Comparing to standard HA, the lack of OH^- ions in OHA's structure brought in the following changes in its *in vitro* behavior: high solubility and partial formation of HA. In addition, the content of incorporated carbonate was not as pronounced as those in immersed HA. These changes mainly resulted from the instability of its structure, because the lack of hydroxyl group leads to a distortion of the hexagonal symmetry. As the OH^- ions are more tightly bound to the surrounding Ca ions than the oxygen-vacancy pair, the substitution of the OH ion by an oxygen-vacancy pair eased the Ca ion release, so that the solubility was increased. The instability of the structure also enabled OHA to have high reactivity with water and be converted into OHA — HA solid solutions. Therefore, the major contribution of — OH to the bioactivity of HA is to provide stability to the hexagonal structure of HA.

Second, consider the *in vitro* behavior of fluorapatite (FAP), which is represented by $Ca_{10}(PO_4)_6F_2$. FAP exhibits hexagonal symmetry. Comparing to the structure of HA, the substitution of F for OH causes a contraction in the *a*-axis dimension, and the crystallinity and stability of the structure were thereby increased. This is reflected on the fact that F-substituted apatites are less soluble than F-free apatites. However, FAP still possesses bioactivity. These findings are in good agreement with the above conclusion that it is the crystallinity and stability of the structure that decide the *in vitro* behavior of materials.

Finally, we may take a look at the structure of hydroxy-carbonate apatite (HCA), which is the product of the *in vitro* reaction. Carbonate, CO_3, can substitute either for the hydroxyl (OH) or the phosphate (PO_4) groups; designated as Type *A* or Type *B* substitutions, respectively. Biological apatite refers to only Type *B* substitutions, which can be expressed by Eq. (7.22)

$$(Ca, \ M)_{10}(PO_4, \ CO_3)_6(OH)_2 \qquad (7.22)$$

where *M* is monovalent ions for charge balance. It is obvious that — OH groups remain untouched, as can be proven further through infrared spectroscopy(IR) spectra of HA before and after the immersion (Fig. 6.10 in Chapter 6). Little change can be found for those peaks at $3,573 \ cm^{-1}$ and $631cm^{-1}$, which were assigned to — OH groups.

7.3   References

1. Verhoeven, J. D. Foundamentals of Physical Metallurgy. John Wiley & Sons, New York (1975)
2. Christofferssen, J., M. R. Christoffersen, J. Cryst. Growth. **57**: 21(1982)
3. Margolis, H. C, E. C. Moreno, Calcif. Tissue. Int. **50**: 137(1992)
4. F. C. M. Driessens. Bioceramics of Calciumphosphate. In: de Groot, K., ed. CRC Press, Boca Raton, FL, p.1(1983)
5. Daculsi, G., R. Z. LeGreros, D. Mitre, Calcif. Tiss. Int. **45**: 95 – 103(1989)
6. Niwa, S., K. Sawai, S. Takahashi, H. Tagai, M. Ono, Y. Fukuda. Appl. Biomat. **2**: 147 – 152(1991)
7. Young, R. A., J. C. Elliot. Archs. Oral. Biol. **11**: 699 – 707(1966)
8. A. E. Nielsen. Industrial crystallization **78**: 159(1979)
9. Burton, W. K, N. Cabrera, Frank, F. C. Phil. Trans. Roy. Soc. pp. 243 – 299 (1951)
10. Kobuko, T., A. Ito, M. Sugiyama, S. Sakka. J. Mater. Sci. **22**: 4067(1987)

7.4   Problems

1. What are the bonding mechanisms of HA film on porous alumina for the coating methods used in this research?
2. What is the deposition mechanism of the HA on porous alumina?
3. Develop a general expression of nucleation and growth.

4. The work of formation, W, for a stable nucleus is the maximum value of the net energy change, ΔG (occurring at r_c). Derive an expression for W in terms of σ and ΔG_v, where σ is the surface free energy and ΔG_v is the volume free energy. (Hint: develop an expression for r_c in terms of σ and ΔG_v first by taking $(d\Delta G/dr)r_c = 0$).

5. Assume heterogeneous nucleation of β forms only in the α-phase (i.e. $A_{\beta\gamma} = A_{\alpha\gamma} = \pi\gamma^2$) and that the area and volume of the spherical cap are given by the equations below ($A_{\alpha\beta}$, V_{cap}). (See Figs. 7.4 and 7.5) Find the critical γ^* (not $\gamma^*\alpha\beta$) and the critical free energy ΔG^* in terms of $\sigma_{\alpha\beta}$ and θ.

$$A_{\alpha\beta} = 2\pi\gamma^2\alpha\beta(1 - \cos\theta)$$
$$V_{\alpha\beta} = 1/3\ \pi\gamma^3\alpha\beta(1 - \cos\theta)^2(2 + \cos\theta)$$
$$f(\theta) = (1 - \cos\theta)^2(2 + \cos\theta)$$

6. How can a flat substrate be "wet" by a liquid and how can you determine the degree at which the substrate is "wet"?

7. Explain the mechanism of bioactivity studied in this research.

8. Is the bioactivity studied in this research a thermally assisted process? If yes, how is the activation energy affected by temperature?

8 Biomedical Metallic Materials[*]

Metals are used as biomedical materials because of their excellent mechanical properties and fair biocompatibility. Metals exhibit excellent strength and resistance to fracture, which are crucial for the medical applications requiring load bearing. Among extensive varieties of metallic materials, a number of them exhibit good biocompatibility, i.e. they do not cause serious toxic reactions in the human body, including stainless steels, cobalt alloys, titanium alloys, and noble metals. The materials for the devices generate less concern in their biocompatibility with human body than those for implants. This chapter introduces metallic materials now being used for medical implants except noble metals in dental applications. The first sections provide basic knowledge of metallurgy that is relevant to implant metals, for those readers who lack background in materials science; later sections describe the production, pros and cons of specific alloys in use and under research.

8.1 Microstructures and Processing

The properties of metallic materials directly derive from their chemical composition and history of thermal and/or mechanical processing — both of which can determine their crystal phase and microstructure. Thus, basic knowledge of metal composition, microstructure and processing is necessary when selecting or developing a metallic material for a specific application.

Crystal Structure

The crystal structures of metals are relatively simple compared with those of ceramics. Three major crystal structures are the body-centered cubic (BCC); face-centered cubic (FCC); and hexagonal close-packed (HCP) as shown in Fig. 8.1. Table 8.1 lists the crystal structures of commonly used metals as engineering materials. Metals with the same crystal structure have certain common features. For example, FCC metals are usually more ductile, i.e. can sustain large plastic deformation without fracture. This is one of the

---

[*] Author is Yang Leng.

main reasons that some FCC metals are used to make dental implants of complex shapes. Note that iron, titanium and cobalt, have more than one type of crystal structure, called as polymorphism. Polymorphic metals readily undergo solid-state phase transformation, from one type to another. For example, steels (iron alloys) include both those with FCC-type structure (austenitic steels) and those with BCC-type structure (ferritic steels). The majority of metallic materials are alloys, not pure metal. Alloys are the metal systems containing more than one designed chemical element. Alloys may contain one or more microscopic constituents with one or more crystal structures. We often name an alloy system according to its main chemical element, such as titanium alloys, cobalt alloys, etc. In an alloy system, crystal structure can be manipulated by varying its chemical composition. For example, increasing nickel content in stainless steels results in FCC type, instead of BCC type stainless steels.

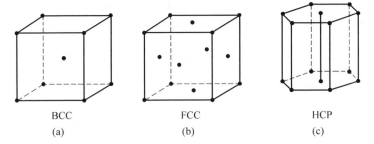

BCC   FCC   HCP

(a)   (b)   (c)

Figure 8. 1 Common crystal structures of metals. (a) body-centered cubic (BCC); (b) face-centered cubic (FCC); and (c) hexagonal close-packed (HCP)

Table 8. 1   Crystal structures of common metals

Metal	Crystal	Metal	Crystal	Metal	Crystal
Aluminum (Al)	FCC	Chromium (Cr)	BCC	Cobalt (Co) ε	HCP
Cobalt (Co) α	FCC	Niobium (Nb)	BCC	Magnesium (Mg)	HCP
Gold (Au)	FCC	Iron (Fe) α	BCC	Titanium (Ti) α	HCP
Copper (Cu)	FCC	Molybdenum (Mo)	BCC	Zinc (Zn)	HCP
Iron (Fe) γ	FCC	Tantalum (Ta)	BCC	Zirconium (Zr)	HCP
Lead (Pb)	FCC	Titanium (Ti) β	BCC		
Nickel (Ni)	FCC	Tungsten (W)	BCC	Manganese (Mn)	Cubic
Platinum (Pt)	FCC	Vanadium (V)	BCC	Tin (Sn)	Tetragonal
Sliver (Ag)	FCC				
Palladium (Pd)	FCC				

Properties of a metallic material, such as its strength, fracture resistance and corrosion resistance, change with its alloying conditions and its history of heat treatment and deformation during metal forming. Thus, we often see that mechanical properties of a metal alloy are specified not only by its chemical composition but also by its conditions of heat treatment and metal forming. For example, mechanically deforming a titanium alloy at ambient temperature can significantly increase its yield strength and tensile strength.

Thermal Treatments

Annealing — Annealing is the process by which metals are heated to an elevated temperature for an extended period and then slowly cooled. The main objective of annealing is to obtain a more thermodynamically stable crystal structure (or phase) or morphology of microscopic features. The functions of annealing include: (a) relieving internal stress generated by plastic deformation and other processing; (b) increasing ductility or toughness, and (c) homogenizing composition and properties. Annealed metals are usually soft and ductile.

Quenching — Quenching is the process by which a meta-stable crystalline phase is obtained by rapidly cooling metals from high to ambient temperature using a cooling medium such as water. Martensite is a typical meta-stable phase produced in steel by quenching. Steels can be hardened by quenching because the martensite of steel is the extremely hard crystalline phase.

Ageing — The function of the aging treatment is to strengthen metal alloys by producing micrometer-scale precipitation (precipitation hardening). Figure 8.2 illustrates the method of aging for precipitation hardening. The aging treatment is effective only with the alloy having a single phase structure at elevated temperatures but a multiple phase structure at ambient temperature. Thus, the alloy have a supersaturated single phase when quenched from a single-phase state at elevated temperatures. Then precipitation of second phase, from the supersaturated solid solution, occurs over an extended time period either at ambient or an elevated temperature within the two-phase region as shown in the phase diagram in Fig. 8.2. An aged alloy exhibits higher strength and lower ductility than its annealed counterpart.

Metal Forming

Casting — Casting metals refers to pouring liquid metal into molds and allowing it to solidify in order to have a specific shape, as schematically shown in Fig. 8.3. It is the simplest way to make metal products with complicated geometry. The molds for casting are commonly made from sand, ceramics, or refractory metals. The investment casting is a technique for making products with high geometric precision. During the process, a mold cavity for a desired shape is firstly produced as a wax pattern. The wax pattern with near final

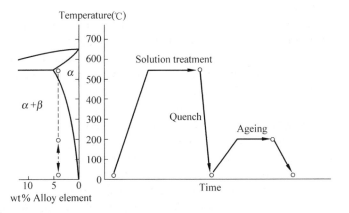

Figure 8.2 The composition requirement and procedure of aging treatment. The alloy composition must be in the range in which solid solubility of the alloy element decreases with decreasing temperature. Precipitates (β-phase) are generated in oversaturated solid solution (α-phase) during aging and results in precipitation strengthening

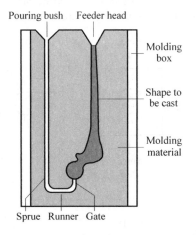

Figure 8.3 Schematic illustration of sand casting. Melted metal is poured into a mold through the sprue, runner and gate. The feeder head is for extra amount of melted metal escape and for feeding cavity caused by shrinkage in cooling

dimensions is then coated with a ceramic shell (investment). After the wax pattern is melted, the metal liquid is poured into the investment, copying the shape of the wax pattern. Casting is a relatively cheap process of metal forming. Casting, however, produces an inhomogeneous microstructure and possible defects such as porosity during solidification. Annealing often is required to

113

improve the properties of casting products.

Cold and Hot Work — Metals can sustain extensive permanent (plastic) deformation by mechanically forming processes such as forging, rolling, extrusion and drawing as illustrated in Fig. 8.4. The mechanical work is applied not only to change shape but also to improve microstructure and mechanical properties. The mechanical work has two types: cold work and hot work defined by the working temperature. The cold working of metal refers to the mechanical deformation at a temperature substantially lower than its melting temperature(TM), usually, less than one-half of its melting temperature (in degrees Kelvin). During cold work, a metal is hardened due to a strain hardening effect. Thus, cold work is widely used as means to increase hardness and strength. Crystal grains of metal may preferentially orient along certain direction in metal, e.g. the rolling direction. Thus, a cold worked metal shows a high level anisotropy of mechanical properties. The hot working of metal refers the mechanical deformation a temperature higher than one-half of its melting temperature (in degrees Kelvin). A wrought metal refers to a metal that has gone through hot working in order to change its original microstructure formed during solidification. Hot work does not generate strain hardening as the cold work does. Its microstructure is usually more homogeneous and stable.

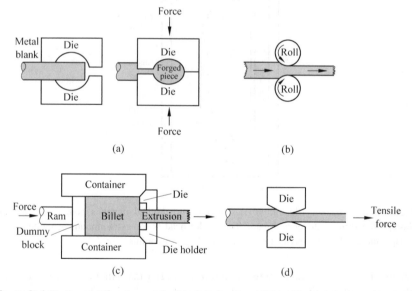

Figure 8.4 Four metal-forming methods. (a) forging; (b) rolling; (c) extrusion; and (d) drawing. (Reprinted from Callister WD, *"Materials Science and Engineering: An Introduction,"* copyright © 2003 by John Wiley & Son, with permission from John Wiley & Sons)

Powder Metallurgy — The powder metallurgy (P/M) is a metal forming process to make products from metal powder. In the processing, metal powder is compacted in a die under high pressure, and then the powder "compact" is heated to a high temperature (lower than its melting point) for a long period of time. This heating process is called sintering. During sintering, the powder particles bond together by extensive mass flow and eventually form a solid product. One of the popular methods is to sinter powder compacts using a hot-isostatic press (HIP). Products of HIP processing are superior to the ones of conventional sintering because HIP effectively enhances bonding between powder particles and reduces porosity of products. Powder metallurgy is in some ways similar to both casting and mechanical working; however, it has two unique features. (1) it can generate metals with more homogenous composition and microstructure; and (2) it can generate alloy systems of chemical composition that cannot be produced by casting because there is no limit on the composition of the mixing powder.

8.2　Corrosion Resistance of Metals

Although having excellent mechanical properties, metallic materials can have serious corrosion problems in aqueous solution, such as in contact with physiological fluids. Corrosion results in releasing toxic metal ions to body and also weakening implants. Thus, corrosion resistance is a primary criterion in selecting metals for biomedical implants. An electrochemical reaction involves removing electrons from the anode to the cathode. Corrosion in physiological environment is an electrochemical reaction involving aqueous body fluid that has dissolved oxygen. The corrosion mechanism in an aqueous solution is schematically illustrated in Fig. 8.5. When a metal is surrounded by an aqueous solution, oxidation may occur at the location on the metal surface, e. g. crevices, where the oxygen concentration in the solution is lower than the normal level. Such location becomes the anode of electrochemical cell where metal molecules lose valence electrons in an oxidation reaction:

$$M \longrightarrow M^{n+} + ne^- \qquad (8.1)$$

In the meantime, electrons move through the metal body to the surface where the concentration of oxygen is higher. That surface becomes the cathode of electrochemical cell where electrons react with oxygen and water molecules to become hydroxyl ions in a reduction reaction:

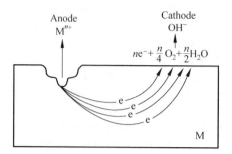

Figure 8.5 Metal corrosion in aqueous solution. Oxidation occurs at the location (anode) where oxygen concentration in solution is low

$$\frac{n}{4}O_2 + \frac{n}{2}H_2O + ne^- \longrightarrow nOH^- \tag{8.2}$$

As a result of oxidation/reduction in physiological fluid, metal ions are released into the body environment and implants gradually lose mechanical integrity. Different metals exhibit different tendency of losing their valence electrons (to be oxidized); the tendency of a metal being oxidized is ranked according to its standard electromotive force (EMF), as shown in Table 8.2. A metal having a higher standard electrode potential is more resistant to losing valence electrons, i.e. it is more resistant to corrosion.

Table 8.2　The standard EMF series

Metal ⟶ Metal Ion	Standard Electrode Potential (V)	
Au ⟶ Au^{3+}	+1.50	
Pt ⟶ Pt^{2+}	+1.2	
Pd ⟶ Pd^{2+}	+0.99	
Ag ⟶ Ag^+	+0.80	
Cu ⟶ Cu^{2+}	+0.34	
H ⟶ H^+	0	Increasingly inert
Ni ⟶ Ni^{2+}	−0.25	
Co ⟶ Co^{2+}	−0.28	Increasingly active
Fe ⟶ Fe^{2+}	−0.44	
Cr ⟶ Cr^{2+}	−0.74	
Al ⟶ Al^{3+}	−1.66	
Ti ⟶ Ti^{3+}	−2.00	
Mg ⟶ Mg^{2+}	−2.36	

When two metals with different EMF potentials are present in a corrosive environment, the metal with higher potential will be the cathode being protected and other will be the anode being corroded. An electrochemical reaction with two different materials acting as anode and cathode, respectively, is called the Galvanic reaction. Thus, having more than one type of metals in an implant should be avoided in order to prevent it from the Galvanic corrosion.

From Table 8.2, we can understand why noble metals are chosen for biomedical applications. Because of their high standard electrode potential, they are basically inert. However, we note that titanium, cobalt and chromium do not have high standard electrode potential, but they are commonly used in biomedical applications. In fact, there are two types of corrosion-resistant materials: (a) those naturally inert, and (b) those that are functionally inert due to the formation of a passive film on surfaces. The passive film is a dense oxide film on the metal surfaces that effectively prevents metal under the surface from oxidation. For example, the corrosion resistance of stainless steel is attributed to chromium oxide film on its surface, and similarly titanium oxide film protects titanium from oxidation. The process of forming the oxide film is called passivation.

8.3 Biological Tolerance of Metal

Corrosion of metal implants in the human body is a primary issue to be concerned because it not only weakens the implant itself, but also risks causing damage to the body, as releasing metal ions into body fluids and tissues. Such corrosion can occur in two ways: (1) physical erosion by wearing (as in artificial joints), and (2) electrochemical corrosion. Our human body contains minute amounts of metallic elements (such as iron, manganese, magnesium, zinc, etc.), which are necessary for normal biological functions. Excessive amounts of such elements however cause toxic reactions. Released metal ions from implants may cause local inflammation, mutations (mutagenesis), or even cancer (carcinogenesis). Table 8.3 provides the tolerances of the human body to the metal elements commonly used in metal implants.

Table 8.3 Metal tolerances in human body

Metal	Normal Amount	Comments
Fe	4 – 5 g in whole body	Element of red blood cells. One of the least toxic trace elements.
Co	Related to B_{12} amount	Element of vitamin B_{12}, No biological function of free Co. May Pure Co is toxic to bone tissue. Co-Cr alloys are not toxic. High dose may be carcinogenic.
Cr	2.8 μg /100 g in blood	Toxic and Affecting cell viability and diminishing DNA synthesis. Hexavalent Cr is carcinogenic.
Mn	12 – 20 mg in whole body	Essential elements in cells. One of the least toxic trace elements.
Mo	1 – 3 ppm in liver	Necessary for certain enzymes to function, Toxic in high dose. Also possible interfere with metabolism of Ca and P.
Ni	5 mg/L in blood	Essential element for limited biological activities. High dose is toxic and may be carcinogenic.
Ag		Not inert in body. Strong inhibitory and bactericidal effects.
Ti		No normal function, but not carcinogenic.
Al		Having adverse effects. Causing deficiencies in bone calcification and neural disorders.
V		Toxic.

8.4 Stainless Steel

Stainless steel, a special type of steel alloy with high resistance to corrosion, has the longest history among metallic materials being used for implants. Its superior resistance to corrosion derives from a dense film of chromium oxide (passive film) that naturally forms on the iron surface. Thus, high content of chromium (at least 11 wt%) is the basic requirement for stainless steel. Other alloys commonly used in stainless steel include nickel, molybdenum and manganese. There are three types of stainless steels, categorized according to their crystalline phase: ferritic, austenitic, and martensitic. Ferritic steels have the BCC crystal structure; austenitic steels have the FCC crystal structure, and martensitic can form a metastable martensitic phase by quenching. Martensitic stainless steels have been used for medical surgery tools. The high strength and high hardness of martensitic stainless steels is necessary for surgery knifes and clips, which cannot be achieved by austenitic ones. The high hardness of martensitic steels is obtained by phase transformation from austenite to martensite by heat treatment. In order to have the martensitic transformation, the carbon content in steel must be sufficiently high. Carbon content in the martensitic stainless steels varies from 0. 15 wt% to 1 wt%. Both ferritic and austenitic steels contain less carbon than martensitic ones. Ferritic steels, while relatively cheap due to low content of expensive nickel, are less corrosion-resistant and less ductile than the austenitic ones. Austenitic steels with the highest corrosion resistance and ductility among stainless steels are universally chosen for medical implants, despite the higher cost. In view of this, the rest of this chapter introduces the properties and development of austenitic steels.

Chemical Composition

Austenitic stainless steels differ from other types in chemical composition. Figure 8. 6 is a composition map of stainless steels in which the domains of ferritic, austenitic and martensitic stainless steel are marked according to their contents of nickel (equivalent) and chromium (equivalent). Figure 8. 6 indicates that about 8 wt% nickel is necessary for austenitic steels with the chromium content of 15 wt%. High concentration of nickel in the austenitic stainless steels stabilizes the FCC phase because the nickel is an FCC crystal itself. Austenitic stainless steels contain a low level of carbon in order have better corrosion resistance, because reducing the carbon content correspondingly reduces

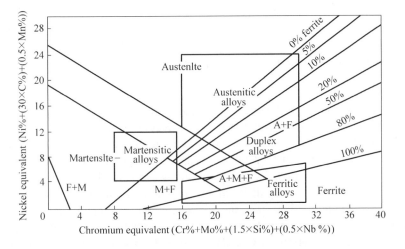

Figure 8. 6 The composition requirements for different types of stainless steels. The nickel and chromium concentrations are expressed to their equivalents in order to account for influence of elements other than nickel and chromium. (Reprinted from Davis JR, *"ASM Special Handbook, Stainless Steels,"* with permission from ASM International)

the formation of carbides such as $Cr_{23}C_6$. Such carbide formation at grain boundaries causes chromium depletion in nearby regions. This is highly undesirable because low chromium in the region near grain boundary diminishes the chromium oxide film for protecting iron from corrosion.

The first stainless steel used for a human implant was 18Cr—8Ni (type 302), which was strong and highly resistant to corrosion. Later, the 18Cr—8Ni was supplemented with a small amount of molybdenum and silicon (type 316), and this became the standard metal alloy for medical implants. The inclusion of molybdenum enhances resistance when chloride ions are present, as is true in body fluids. In the 1950s, a low carbon version of 316 (type 316L) was developed to reduce the carbon content from 0.08 wt% to 0.03 wt% in order to improve corrosion resistance further. Table 8.4 lists compositions of various austenitic steels used for medical implants. While many alloys have been tried, 316L is still the stainless steel most commonly used for manufacturing medical implants.

Table 8.4   Nominal composition of austenitic steels for medical implants (wt%)

Type (AISI number) *	Fe	C (max)	Cr	Ni	Mo	Mn
302	bal	0.15	18	9	...	2.0
304	bal	0.08	19	9	...	2.0
316	bal	0.08	17	12	2.5	2.0
316L	bal	0.03	17	12	2.5	2.0

* AISI stands for American Iron and Steel Institute.

Microstructure

Two microstructure features of an austenitic stainless steel, affecting its performance, are grain size and shape. The recommended grain size for 316L is 100 μm or less. Generally, the smaller the grains, the stronger and tougher the steel is. Because smaller grains means more grain boundaries, and the grain boundaries provide resistance to plastic deformation because they are barriers for slip deformation by dislocations. A relation between yield strength and grain size is quantified as that the yield strength is proportional to $1/d^{1/2}$, where d is the average grain diameter (Hall-Patch relation). The American society for testing and materials (ASTM) grades the grain size by numbers, where higher numbers correspond to smaller grains. For example, #6 means a grain size of about 100 μm.

Shape of austenitic steel grains depends on processing history. Under an annealed condition, austenite grains of the stainless steel have an equiaxial granular shape , as shown in Fig. 8.7. However , in a cold - worked condition, the grains might be elongated (i.e. longer in the rolling direction), depending on the amount of cold work. Large plastic deformation causes grains to rotate and results in a textured grain structure in which grains preferentially align themselves in certain crystallographic orientations (see Fig. 8.8). Thus, a cold-worked stainless steel with textured structure exhibits anisotropic mechanical properties. Microstructure examination is recommended when using a cold-worked stainless steel for implant manufacturing because implants can be better made if the loading direction is parallel to the high strength direction in the steels.

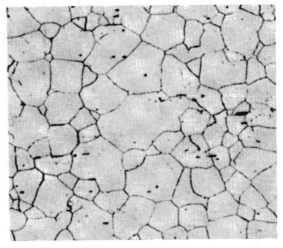

Figure 8.7 Optical micrograph of annealed 316 austenitic stainless steel exhibiting equiaxed grains. (Reprinted from Davis JR, *"ASM Special Handbook, Stainless Steels,"* with permission from ASM International)

Mechanical Properties

The low carbon content of austenitic stainless steel prevents it from being hardened by heat treatment, i.e. it is not heat treatable. Instead, cold working is often used to increase mechanical strength. Cold working produces plastic deformation in the steels and generates a strain hardening effect, which improves both yield strength and tensile strength of stainless steel substantially. The amount of cold work is commonly defined as a percentage of cross-section area reduction by plastic deformation; in the figures in this chapter, it is indicated as "cold reduction". For example, if cold working reduces a metal bar with cross section of 100 mm × 20 mm to a cross section of 100 mm × 10 mm, then the cold reduction is 50%. Figure 8.9 illustrates the effects of strain hardening on mechanical properties of type 316L. Note that the ductility

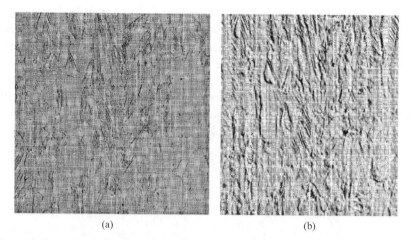

(a)　　　　　　　　　　　　　　　(b)

Figure 8.8 Optical micrographs of cold-worked 316L austenitic stainless steel. Revealing microstructure of the 316 type of stainless steels could be difficult in metallography due to its high resistance to chemical etching. Figure 8.8(b) is the micrograph obtained by differential interference contrast, which reveals the features better than that of bright field one (Fig. 8.8(a)). (Reprinted from Davis JR, "*ASM Special Handbook, Stainless Steels,*" with permission from ASM International)

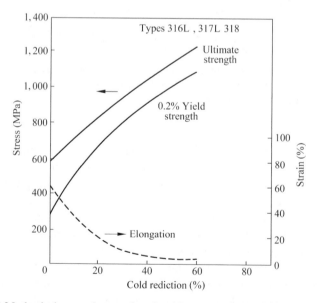

Figure 8.9 Mechanical properties as a function of amount of cold work in stainless steels. Cold reduction refers to the percentage of cold work (ASTM 1980)

of the stainless steels is scarificed to a certain extent at the expense of strengthening. Since the extent of cold working determines, to a great extent, the properties of austenitic stainless steels, attention must be paid to the amount of cold work when selecting steels for a particular purpose. Table 8.5 lists the mechanical properties data of 316 and 316L in annealed and cold worked conditions.

Table 8.5   Mechanical properties of 316 and 316L stainless steels

Type	Treatment Condition	Young's Modulus (GPa)	Yield Strength (MPa)	Tensile Strength (MPa)	Ductility (% elongation)
316L*	Annealed	190	172	485	40
	Cold worked	190	690	860	12
316	Annealed	190	205	515	40
	Cold worked	190	690	860	12

* 316L data are from ASTM F139-86, p. 61 1992. The ASTM code of 316L is F138 or F139. ASTM Committee F-4 on Surgical Implant Materials has written standard specifications for the metals using for implants. Thus specifications are designated as letter F followed by 1 to 3 integers.

8.5   Cobalt-Based Alloys

Cobalt-based alloys have even better corrosion resistance in physiological environments than stainless steels. The cobalt alloys are also more wear resistant than stainless steels, even though they are heavier.

Chemical Composition

The cobalt-based alloys for implants are derived from Co—Cr or Co—Ni—Cr system with high strength and high corrosion resistance. There are three alloys commonly used for medical implants: cast or P/M Co—Cr—Mo (F75 or Stellite 21); wrought Co—Cr—W—Ni (F90 or Stellite 25); and Co—Ni—Cr—Mo—Ti (F562 or MP35N). All the medical grade Co-based alloys are the low-carbon types (= 0.25 wt%), and the rest of their compositions are listed in Table 8.6.

Table 8.6 Compositions of cobalt-based alloys for biomedical implants (wt%)

Alloys	ASTM Designation	Co	Cr	Mo	W	Ni	Fe	Si	Mn
Cast or P/M Co—Cr—Mo	F75	Bal	27.0 – 30.0	5.0 – 7.0	...	2.75	0.75	1.0	1.0
Wrought Co—Cr—W—Ni	F90	Bal	19.0 – 21.0	...	14.0 – 16.0	9.0 – 11.0	3 (max)	0.4	1.0 – 2.0
Wrought Co—Ni—Cr—Mo	F562	Bal	19.0 – 21.0	9.0 – 10.5	...	33.0 – 37.0	1 (max)	0.15 (max)	0.15 (max)

In F75 and F90, cobalt and chromium form solid solutions (ε-Co) in the alloys as shown in the Co—Cr phase diagram (Fig. 8.10). Chromium increases corrosion resistance and provides solid solution strengthening. Molybdenum is added to produce finer grains and strengthen the solid solution. In F90, tungsten and nickel are added to improve machinability and fabrication properties. F75 (Stellite 21) is primarily designed for making implants by the investment casting. F562 is a multiphase alloy with a large amount of nickel, which stabilizes the FCC solid solution phase (α-Co). Such composition ensures that it can be strengthened by the solid-state phase transformation from FCC (α) to

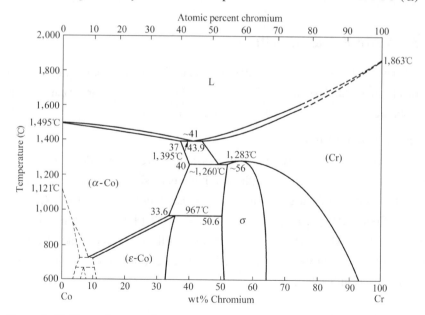

Figure 8.10 Phase diagram of a cobalt-chromium system (Reprinted from Davis JR, "*ASM Special Handbook, Stainless Steels,*" with permission from ASM International)

hexagonal close-packed (HCP) (ε) structure during cold working, and it can further strengthen Co_3Mo precipitation by a subsequent aging.

Microstructure

Microstructure of biomedical cobalt alloys varies significantly with processing conditions. Fig. 8.11(a) shows the typical casting microstructure of the cast F75 alloy which, consists of the Co-rich ε-phase (light background) with interdendritic carbides (dark areas). The solidification process also generates relatively large grains, which is undesirable because of their low mechanical strength. Hot forging produces a wrought alloy in which the microstructure is been modified as shown in Fig. 8.11(b). Refinements of grains and carbides in F75 are achieved by hot forging, and results in improvement of mechanical strength. The F562 consists of fine grains of FCC phase and HCP platelets as shown in Fig. 8.12. Such microstructure indicates high strength of this multiphase alloys resulting from the solid solution strengthening, the grain and/or phase boundary strengthening and the precipitation strengthening after cold working and aging.

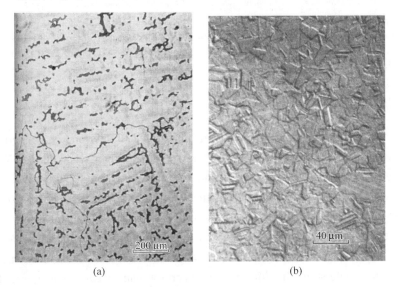

(a)   (b)

Figure 8.11 Microstructure of cobalt-based alloy F75. (a) micrograph of casting microstructure; (b) micrograph of wrought microstructure by interference contrast. (Reprinted from Davis JR, "*ASM Special Handbook, Nickel, Cobalt, and Their Alloys,*" with permission from ASM International.)

Figure 8.12 Microstructure of cobaltk-based alloy F562. The equiaxed FCC grains mix with the dark HCP platelets. (Reprinted from B. D. Ratner et al., *"Biomaterials Science: Introduction to Materials in Medicine,"* copyright © 1996, by Academic Press, with permission from Elsevier)

Mechanical Properties

Generally, the cobalt-based alloys exhibit higher Young's modulus and strength than stainless steel, though their ductility is slightly poorer. Importantly, cobalt-based alloys exhibit better wear resistance than other alloys. Wear resistance of metallic materials relates to their hardness, and hardness increases with yield strength and tensile strength. The high wear resistance of cobalt-based alloys can be demonstrated by their strengths as shown in Table 8.7. The strengths of cobalt-based alloys are highly sensitive to processing conditions. F799, which is the hot forged version of F75, exhibits much higher yield and tensile strength with improved ductility than its cast counterpart. The cold-working effectively strengthens F90 as indicated in the table. The cold working plus aging is more effective than cold working alone to strengthen the multiphase alloy F562 as shown in Fig. 8.13.

Table 8.7   Mechanical properties of cobalt-based alloys for medical implants

Alloys	Treatment Condition	ASTM Designation	Young's Modulus (GPa)	Yield Strength (MPa)	Tensile Strength (MPa)	Ductility (% elongation)
Co—Cr—Mo	Cast	F75	248	450	655	8
Co—Cr—Mo	Wrought	F799	⋯	827	1,172	12
Co—Cr—W—Ni	Wrought	F90	242	379	896	⋯
	44% Cold worked	F90	⋯	1,606	1,896	⋯
Co—Ni—Cr—Mo	Annealed	F562	228	241 − 448	793 − 1,000	50
	Cold worked and aged	F562	⋯	1,586	1,793	8

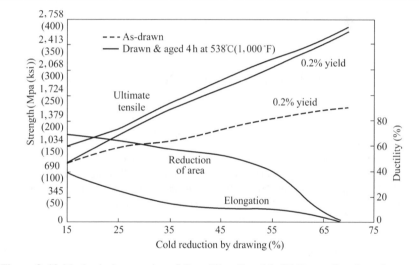

Figure 8.13 Mechanical properties of Co—Ni—Cr—Mo F562 as a function of amount of cold work. (Reprinted from Davis JR, "*ASM Special Handbook, Nickel, Cobalt, and Their Alloys,*" with permission from ASM International.)

8.6   Titanium and Its Alloys

Titanium and its alloys have been increasingly used in medical implants because of their excellent biocompatibility, corrosion resistance and relatively low density. Like stainless steels, titanium alloys form passive films on their surfaces − in this case a TiO_2 film that is the source of their corrosion resistance. Like iron, titanium is polymorphic. As the schematic phase diagram shows (Fig.

127

8.14), low temperature phase of titanium alloys is α-Ti with the HCP crystal structure and the high temperature phase is β - Ti with the BCC crystal structure. At ambient temperature, we can have the α-Ti single phases, or the $\alpha + \beta$ two phases, and even the β-Ti single phase titanium alloys, depending on the alloy's chemical composition. Elements that have been used to stabilize the α-phase include aluminum and tin. Elements that can stabilize the β-phase include vanadium molybdenum, chromium and niobium.

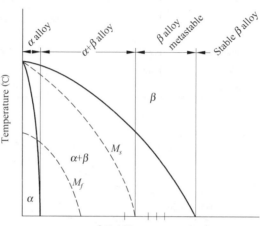

β-Stabilizer concentration

Figure 8.14 Schematic phase diagram of titanium alloy. High contents of β stabilizing elements such as vanadium, niobium will produce $\alpha + \beta$ phase alloy such as Ti -6Al-4V. The M_s and M_f represent the martensitic transformation starting and finishing temperature, respectively. (Reprinted from Matthew JD, "*Titanium, A Technical Guide,*" 2nd edition, with permission from ASM International.)

Chemical Composition

Unalloyed titanium, known as commercially pure (CP), is commonly used titanium material for implants because it is the most corrosion-resistant. Ti CP has four grades according to its trace element content. Grade 4 (Ti CP-4) has the highest level of trace elements of oxygen, iron and carbon. Such elements are called the interstitial elements in titanium because they form interstitial solid solutions. The titanium alloys are named by their composition, e. g. Ti -6Al-4V contains 6 wt% aluminum and 4 wt% vanadium. Ti -6Al-4V is the $\alpha + \beta$ alloy and the most widely used titanium alloy because of its high strength. Medical grade Ti -6Al-4V has extremely low content of interstitial (ELI) elements. A relatively new $\alpha + \beta$ alloy, Ti -13Nb-13Zr, uses niobium as β-phase stabilizer, and exhibits an interestingly low elastic modulus.

The impurities such as interstitial elements significantly affect mechanical properties of titanium and its alloys. Thus, their contents are tightly controlled during manufacturing as specified in Table 8.8.

Table 8.8   Impurity contents of Ti and Ti alloys for biomedical implants (wt%)

Alloys	ASTM Designation	Ti	C (max)	Fe (max)	H (max)	N (max)	O (max)
TiCP-4	F67	Bal	0.10	0.50	0.015	0.05	0.40
Ti – 6Al – 4V ELI	F136	Bal	0.10	0.20	0.015	0.03	0.13
Ti – 13Nb – 13Zr	F1713	Bal	0.08	0.10	0.02	0.01	0.10

Microstructure

The typical pure titanium used for medical implants is the mildly cold-worked Ti CP. Its microstructure consists of single-phase α-Ti grains (Fig. 8.15). The grain size varies from 10 to 150 μm depending on processing conditions. In contrast, Ti – 6Al – 4V consists of 90 vol% of α-Ti and 10 vol% of β-Ti. Its microstructure can be dramatically changed by treatment. Slow cooling from a single β region generates the microstructure of α-phase platelets (acicular structure) separated by β-phase (Fig. 8.16(a)). Fast cooling can generate a martensite phase (indicated by the M_s and M_f line in Fig. 8.14). The martensite phase grains also have an acicular structure and differentiating them from the α-phase grains is difficult. Forging or rolling at a two-phase temperature produces an equiaxed grain structure (Fig. 8.16(b)). This equiaxed structure is also called "recrystallization-annealed" because the original acicular α-phase grains are replaced by granular ones during a recrystallization annealing after the cold working. Such microstructure improves fatigue resistance of the alloy.

Mechanical Properties

Mechanical properties of the titanium alloys are summarized in Table 8.9. Mechanical properties of Ti CP depend on the conditions of cold working and annealing for a given grade of interstitial element levels. Fully annealed Ti CP-4 with equiaxed grains exhibits lower strength than the cold-worked ones. The mechanical properties of Ti – 6Al – 4V with equiaxed α-phase grains exhibit higher strength and ductility than those with the acicular grains. However, the acicular structure increases resistance to fracture or cracking (i.e. high fracture toughness). Its casting counterpart is inferior in mechanical properties as shown in Table 8.9. Note that Ti – 13Nb – 13Zr exhibits low Young's modulus while maintaining the same strength as Ti – 6Al – 4V. Low Young's modulus is

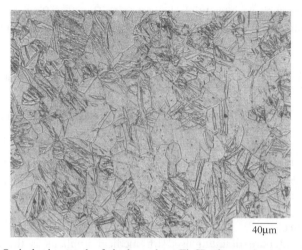

Figure 8.15 Optical micrograph of single α-phase Ti CP after moderately amount of cold working (Reprinted from B. D. Ratner et al., *"Biomaterials Science: Introduction to Materials in Medicine,"* copyright © 1996, by Academic Press, with permission from Elsevier)

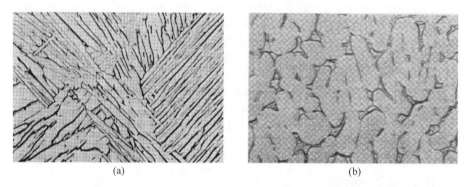

(a)   (b)

Figure 8.16 Optical micrographs of α-β Ti alloy microstructure. (a) microstructure of slow cooling from a single β-phase temperature; (b) microstructure of annealing after hot working. (Reprinted from Matthew JD, *"Titanium, A Technical Guide,"* 2nd edition, with permission from ASM International.)

favorable in medical implants because it reduces the level of stiffness mismatch between bones and implants. The stiffness mismatch between implants and bone can cause a stress shielding effect by which the bone is prevented from load bearing. This effect should be avoided or reduced to a minimum because it causes bone weakening. We should also note that titanium and its alloys commonly exhibit poor resistance to shear stress, comparing with the stainless steels and the cobalt alloys.

Table 8.9 Mechanical properties of Ti and Ti alloys for medical implants

Alloys	Treatment Condition	ASTM Designation	Young's Modulus (GPa)	Yield Strength (MPa)	Tensile Strength (MPa)	Ductility (% elongation)
Ti CP-4	Annealed	F67	110	480	550	15
Ti – 6Al – 4V ELI	Forged and annealed	F136	110	825	890	14
	Casting		110	758	827	13
Ti – 13Nb – 13Zr	Aged	F1713	79	725	860	8

8.7　TiNi Shape Memory Alloy

TiNi is an intermetallic compound with stoichiometric composition (50 at % Ni), which exhibits a special shape memory effect (SME), and pseudoelasticity (PE) or superelasticity (SE). The shape memory phenomenon was discovered in this alloy in the Naval Ordnance Laboratory (NOL), and is thus named Nitinol. There are increasing numbers of applications of Nitinol in medicine because of its advantages for correcting teeth shape (orthodontic dental archwires), expanding blood vessels (vascular stents), etc. Nitinol also exhibits excellent biocompatibility, corrosion resistance and wear resistance.

Shape Memory and Pseudoelasticity

The shape memory effect (SME) of an alloy refers to its ability to recover its original shape at a higher temperature after being deformed beyond its elastic limit at a lower temperature. The SME effect originates from solid-state phase transformation between austenite (a high temperature phase) and martensite (a low temperature phase). Since austenite and martensite have different crystalline structures and density, the transformation from austenite to martensite should result in macroscopically geometric changes. For a shape memory alloy (SMA), as schematically illustrated in Fig. 8.17, the martensite consists of individual domains called variants (marked as A, B, C and D in Fig. 8.17 (b)). The variants are arranged in a manner (self-accommodating) such that the possible geometry change by phase transformation from austenite to martensite is minimized. When the martensite is under deformation, the variants with orientation that favors greater elongation in the direction of the tensile load will grow and other variants will reorient themselves to adopt the deformation

(Fig. 8.17(c)). The strain in variants is recoverable when the SMA is heated up to the point where martensite is transformed to austenite.

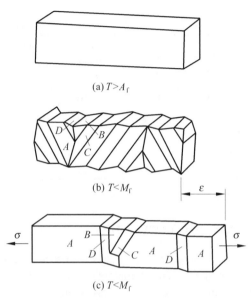

(a) $T>A_f$

(b) $T<M_f$

ε

(c) $T<M_f$

Figure 8.17 Schematic illustration of transformation and deformation in SMA. (a) Original shape in austenite; (b) Shape of martensite in which variants arrangement maintains the original shape; (c) During deformation, variant A in martensite with preferential deformation direction parallel to external stress grows (Reprinted from Brunette DM, Tengvall R, Textor M, Thomsen P, "*Titanium in Medicine,*" with persimssion from Springer-Verlag.)

The pseudoelasticity (PE), also called superelasticity (SE), of an alloy refers to its ability to recover its original shape after the SMA has been deformed beyond its elastic limit (~ 6 % in TiNi) when mechanical force is released. The difference between PE and SME is that PE requires deformation at a temperature higher than that of martensitic transformation (M_s), because the PE requires a stress-induced martensitic transform (SMIT). The stress- induced martensite produces a variant that generates the greatest shape change in the direction of the applied load. Similar to SME, the strain in the variant is recoverable when the applied load releases and the martensite changes back to austenite. Figure 8.18 shows a typical stress/strain curves of SMA in the PE state.

The SME and PE behavior is stress- and temperature-dependent, as schematically illustrated in Fig. 8.19. SME occurs at the temperatures lower

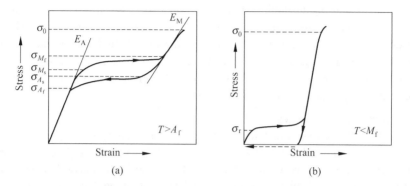

Figure 8.18 Schematic stress/strain curves of a SMA. The arrows indicate either loading or unloading paths. σ_0 represents the critical stress of plastic deformation by dislocation slip. (a) deformation in austenitic phase. The initial slope (E_A) represents the Young's modulus of austenitic phase. The low modulus region is pseudoelastic deformation. After pseudoelastic deformation, the second slope (E_M) represent the Young's modulus of martensitic phase; (b) deformation in martensitic phase. σ_r represents the critical stress of starting variant reorientation. The deformation generated by variant reorientation in martensite can be fully recovered at a temperature higher than A_f(Reprinted from Brunette DM, Tengvall R, Textor M, Thomsen P, "*Titanium in Medicine,*" with persimssion from Springer-Verlag.)

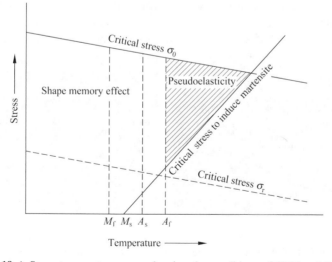

Figure 8.19 A Stress-temperature map, showing the conditions of SME and PE. σ_f represents the critical stress for reorientation of martensite variants. σ_0 represents the critical stress for plastic deformation by dislocation ship

than that of starting austenitic transformation (A_s) and at stress levels higher than the critical stress required for reorienting martensite variants. While PE occurs at the temperatures above A_f and at stress levels higher than those critical for SIMT. At a temperature between A_s and A_f, SME and PE can only partially occur. The upper bound of the SME and PE represents the critical stress for conventional plastic deformation by dislocation slip.

Structure and Properties

TiNi SMA has an equiatomic or near-equiatomic composition ($50\% - 50.5\%$ Ni). The austenite phase in TiNi is an ordered CsCl or B2-type crystal structure. There are two martensitic phases in TiNi, the rhombohedral R-phase and the monoclinic B19' phase. Thermo-mechanical treatment induces a two-step transformation in TiNi, $B2 \rightarrow R \rightarrow B19'$.

The SME and PE of TiNi are sensitive to thermo-mechanical treatments. Figure 8.20 shows the TiNi microstructure in different annealing conditions after 25% cold rolling. A full annealing generates recrystallization from cold worked grains, and forms stress-free grains as shown in Fig. 8.20(a), while low temperature annealing retains deformed grains and yields a microstructure as shown in Fig. 8.20(b). The recrystallization annealing (full annealing) reduces the TiNi resistance to dislocation slip and causes partial SME and PE as shown in Fig. 8.21(a). SME and PE are improved by annealing below the crystallization temperature (873 K) as shown in Fig. 8.21(b), because the TiNi retains the strengthening of cold work. SME and PE can be improved by other strengthening methods, such as increasing the amount of cold work and decreasing grain size. On the other hand, lowering deformation temperature is also

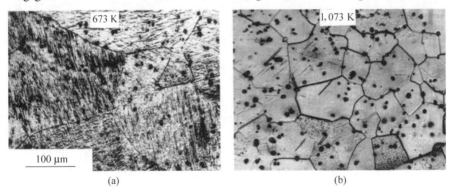

(a)   (b)

Figure 8.20 Optical micrographs of 25% cold-worked TiNi annealed at (a) 400°C; and (b) 800°C. (Reprinted from Otsuka K, Wayman CM, *"Shape Memory Materials,"* with persimssion from Cambridge University Press.)

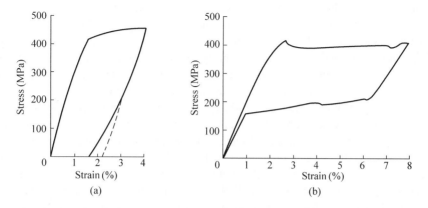

Figure 8.21 Stress/strain curves of 25% cold-worked TiNi loaded at 60°C. (a) after annealing at 850°C, the PE is indicated by the difference between the dash line and solid line of unload curve. The arrow indicates the level of SME. (b) after annealing at 400°C, PE completely recovers the deformation. (Reprinted from Otsuka K, Wayman CM, *"Shape Memory Materials,"* with persimssion from Cambridge University Press.)

good for SME because of higher critical stress of dislocation slip as shown in Fig. 8.19.

Certain medical applications require shape recovery at about body temperature. TiNi with stoichiometric composition (50% Ni) has the highest shape recovery temperature (about 120°C). This temperature decreases with increase of Ni concentration in the binary TiNi. Additions of alloy elements also can effectively change the transformation temperatures, and thus the shape recovery temperature. Substitution of cobalt and iron for nickel lowers the transformation temperature. Substitution of vanadium, chromium and manganese for titanium also lowers the transformation temperature. The transformation temperature is sensitive to concentrations of oxygen and carbon in TiNi. Oxygen and carbon consume titanium to form Ti_4Ni_2O and TiC. Such oxide formation in TiNi effectively changes the ratio of Ti and results in lowering the transformation temperature. Sensitivity of TiNi SME and PE to compositions as well as treatment conditions provides selections for specific biomedical applications.

8.8 Summary

In summary, their excellent mechanical properties make metallic materials unique among the implant materials. Table 8.10 compares the mechanical properties of metal systems for medical implants. A remarkable feature of metallic materials is that their mechanical properties are sensitive to processing and heat treatment. This feature enables us to manipulate them, without the need to change their chemical compositions to suit specific applications in surgery. Corrosion resistance and biocompatibility limit our selections to only several metal systems discussed in this chapter. Among the materials listed in Table 8.10, titanium system stands out as the top choice because of its excellent bio-compatibility, while stainless steels have traditionally wide applications because of economic reasons. Cobalt-based alloys are more commonly used in implants requiring high wear resistance. Table 8.11 lists current applications of stainless steels, cobalt alloys, titanium alloys and Ti — Ni shape memory alloys in surgery. The applications of metallic materials have been increasing, and are not necessarily limited to those in Table 8.11. Although new biomaterials are being developed, metallic materials continuously play a major role as the materials of orthopedic and dental implants.

Table 8.10   Property comparison of metallic materials for biomedical implants

Alloys	Density (g/cm^3)	Young's Modulus (GPa)	Yield Strength (MPa)	Corrosion Resistance*
Ti and its alloys	4.5	79 – 116	485 – 1,034	+ + +
Stainless steel (316L)	7.9	190	221 – 1,213	+
Co-based alloys	8.3 – 9.2	210 – 253	448 – 1,500	+ + + +
TiNi SMA	6.7	~ 60**	...	+ +

* Higher number of " + " sign presents better corrosion resistance.   ** in austenite phase.

Table 8.11   Summary of metallic materials for medical implants

Applications	Metals
Orthopedics	
Bone plates	Stainless steels, Titanium alloys
Screws	Stainless steels, Cobalt-based alloys, Titanium alloys
Intramedullary pins	Stainless steels
Hip joint	Stainless steels, Cobalt-based alloys, Titanium alloys
Knee joint	Stainless steels, Cobalt-based alloys
Spine disc cages	Stainless steel, Titanium alloys
Rods for scoliosis correction	TiNi shape memory alloys
Dentistry	
Inlay, Crowns, Bridges	Noble-based, Sliver-based, and Nickel-based alloys

Continued

Applications	Metals
Root form implants	Titanium alloys
Blade implants	Stainless steels, Titanium alloys
Subperiosteal implants	Cobalt-based alloys
Ramus frame implants	Stainless steels, Titanium alloys
Arch wire	Stainless steels, TiNi shape memory alloys
Cardiology	
Heart valves	Cobalt-based alloys, TiNi shape memory alloys
Vascular stents	Stainless steels, Cobalt-based alloys, TiNi shape memory alloys
Cardiac pacemaker	Titanium alloys

8.9 References

1. Ratner, B. D., A. S. Hoffman, F. J. Schoen, J. E. Lemons. Biomaterials Science. Academic Press, San Diego (1996)
2. Nicholson, J. W. The Chemistry of Medical and Dental Materials, RSC Materials Monographs. Royal Society of Chemistry, Cambridge (2002)
3. Silver, F. H., D. L. Christiansen. Biomaterials Science and Biocompatibility. Springer, New York (1999)
4. Combe, E. C., F. J. Trevor Burke, W. H. Douglas. Dental Materials. Kluwer Academic Publishers, Boston (1999)
5. Park, J. B., J. D. Bronzino. Biomaterials-Principles and Applications. CRC Press, Boca Raton (2002)
6. Bhat, S. V. Biomaterials. Kluwer Academic Publishers, Boston (2002)
7. Brunette, D. M., R. Tengvall, M. Textor, P. Thomsen. Titanium in Medicine. Springer-Verlag, Berlin (2001)
8. Fontana, M. G. Corrosion Engineering, 3rd edition. McGraw-Hill, New York (1986)
9. Smith, W. F. Structure and Properties of Engineering Alloys, 2nd edition, McGraw-Hill, New York (1993)
10. Davis, J. R. ASM Special Handbook, Stainless Steels. ASM International, Materials Park, Ohio(1994)
11. Davis, J. R. ASM Special Handbook, Nickel, Cobalt, and Their Alloys. ASM International, Materials Park, Ohio (2000)
12. Matthew, J. D. Titanium A Technical Guide, 2nd edition. ASM International, Materials Park, Ohio (2000)
13. Brunette, D. M. R. Tengvall, M. Textor, P. Thomsen. Titanium in Medicine. Springer-Verlag Berlin (2001)
14. Otsuka, K., C. M. Wayman. Shape Memory Materials. Cambridge University Press,

Cambridge, UK (1998)

8.10   Problems

1.   Which material in Table 8.11 is more suitable for shaping an implant by mechanical work at ambient temperature, considering their nature of crystal structure shown in Table 8.1? Why?

2.   Can water be a corrosive environment? If so, how can we make water less corrosive?

3.   Comparing an implant made by (a) cobalt-nickel alloy and stainless steel; and (b) stainless steel only. Which one is more likely to corrode faster? Why?

4.   Why 316L is more favorable for implants than 316?

5.   An implant requires that yield strength is not less than 500 MPa and ductility is not less than 20%. Select a stainless steel with appropriate processing conditions for such implant.

6.   Both wrought and casting Ti −6Al −4VELI are used for making implants. Compare the pros and cons of each type.

7.   Casting titanium alloys are often treated by hot isostatic pressing (HIP). What is the benefit of the HIP treatment?

8.   Hip joints have been made by stainless steel, cobalt-based alloy and titanium alloy. If you are an orthopedic surgeon, which material will you use? Justify your decision.

9.   Select a cobalt-based alloy with appropriate conditions for knee joint implants. Justify your decision.

10.   Arch wires made by TiNi are used to correct the arrangement of teeth by dentists. What the feature (effect) of TiNi are employed to generate consistent pressure on teeth for a long period of time?

Part II

Polymeric Biomaterials[*]

---

* Author of Part II is Qing Lin.

Biomaterials have been widely used in:

(1) orthopedics — joint replacements (hip, knee), bone cements, bone void fillers, fracture fixation plates, and artificial tendons and ligaments;

(2) cardiovascular — vascular grafts, heart valves, pacemakers, artificial heart and ventricular assist device components, stents, balloons, and blood substitutes;

(3) ophthalmics — contact lenses, corneal implants and artificial corneas, and intraocular lenses;

(4) other applications — dental implants, cochlear implants, tissue screws and tacks, burn and wound dressings and artificial skin, tissue adhesives and sealants, drug-delivery systems, matrices for cell encapsulation and (TE), and sutures.

The types of biomaterials used in the above applications include metals (stainless steel, titanium, cobalt chrome), ceramics and glasses (alumina, calcium phosphate, Bioglass^{TM}), and a wide range of synthetic and natural polymers. This part will primarily focus on polymers, and presents a brief overview of the basics of polymer science, some of which expand the capabilities of polymeric biomaterials.

In Chapter 9, some of the basics of the polymeric biomaterials are introduced, such as the characteristics of polymers, types of polymerization to prepare polymers, etc. Then the different types of polymer biomaterials were further discussed in the following chapters, with their specific examples in biomedical applications.

Naturally occurring polymers, such as collagen, chitin and alginate, are an important class of biomaterials because of their biodegradation characteristics and they are rich in resources. Their structures and properties, biomedical applications and chemical modifications methods are summarized in Chapter 10.

Synthetic polymers represent the majority of the polymer biomaterials — from traditional engineering plastics to newly engineered biomaterials for specific biomedical applications. Although most synthetic non-biodegradable polymers are these originally designed for non-biomedical use, they are widely used as biomaterials mainly because of the necessary physical-mechanical properties they have. There are still no newly engineered biomaterials that can replace those non-degradable polymers. A good example is that PMMA bone cement which has been used for the fixation of artificial joint since 1943 and is still being widely used clinically nowadays. These non-biodegradable polymers are reviewed in Chapter 11.

Synthetic biodegradable polymers has attracted much attention in the last decade because the biodegradable polymers can be eliminated from the body after fulfilling their intended use and therefore the second surgery can be avoided. Also, the emerging of tissue engineering has demanded the use of biodegradable scaffolds for the regeneration of tissues and organs. A lot of biodegradable polymers were derived from the traditional polymers by introducing non-stable chemical linkages, such as hydrolysable ester bonds. The biodegradation mechanisms and polymers are summarized in Chapter 12.

The application of biomaterials in orthopedic field represents a significant challenge to the biomaterials scientists. Biomaterials for orthopedic use will have to possess sufficient mechanical properties to share or bear the load, and will also need to be able to bond to host bone. If possible, the biomaterials have to be gradually replaced by newly formed bone. One solution will be to use bioactive ceramics, such as calcium phosphate and Bioglass™, to reinforce polymers so that the mechanical properties and bone bonding properties of the polymer can be improved. Chapter 13 reviews the recent advances in polymer/ceramic composites.

9 Polymer Basics

Polymers are long chain molecules with a wide range of physical and chemical properties. One of the main advantages of the polymer materials is the ease of fabrication to produce various shapes (rod, film, fiber, sheet, etc.). The advances in polymer chemistry have made it possible to tailor the properties of polymers for specific application.

The objective of this chapter is to introduce the readers some basic knowledge of polymers, including the classification of polymers, some characteristics of polymers, and the commonly used reactions for the synthesis of polymers.

9.1 Classification of Polymers

Polymers can be classified according to their sources, chain structures, thermal behaviors, stabilities, etc., as discussed below.

9.1.1 Source

By source, polymers can be divided into two groups. They are naturally occurring polymers and synthetic polymers.

Table 9.1 listed some examples of naturally occurring polymers.

Table 9.1 Commonly seen naturally occurring polymers

	Polymer	Source
A. Proteins	Collagen	Animals
	Silk	Animals
	Keratin	Animals
	Fibrinogen	Animals
	Elastin	Animals

Continued

	Polymer	Source
B. Polysaccharides	Cellulose	Plants
	Starch	Plants
	Chitin	Animals
	Alginic	Brown Seaweeds
	Agar	Red seaweeds

Synthetic polymers are synthesized via polymerization reaction using monomers. The polymerization will be discussed later in Sec. 9.2. Some of the commonly used polymers are listed in Table 9.2.

Table 9.2 Commonly seen synthetic non-biodegradable polymers

Type of Polymer	Name of Polymer	Polymerization Mechanism
Polyolefin	Polyethylene	Radical, ionic chain-reaction polymerization
	Polypropylene	Ionic chain-reaction polymerization
Polyacrylate	Poly(methyl methacrylate)	Radical polymerization
Polyamide	Nylon 66	Step polymerization
	Nylon 6	Step polymerization
Polyurethane	Poly(ether-urethane)	Step polymerization
	Polyester-urethane	Step polymerization
Polyester	Poly(ethylene terephthalate)	Step polymerization
	Poly(butylene terephthalate)	Step polymerization
Polycarbonate	Bisphenol a polycarbonate	Step polymerization
Poly(ether ether ketone)	Poly(ether ether ketone)	Step polymerization
Polysulfones	Polysulfones	Step polymerization

9.1.2 Polymer Chain Structure

According to the backbone structure of the polymer, the polymer can be classified as linear, branched and crosslinked polymers.

9.1.2.1 Linear Polymer

A linear polymer has the following backbone structure (Fig. 9.1).

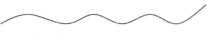

Figure 9.1 Linear polymer chain

For a linear polymer, there are no chemical bonds between each polymer molecular chains. When heated or under stress, the molecular chains can move relatively to each other. Linear polymer can be dissolved in suitable solvents. When heated, the polymer can be molten. Therefore, linear polymers usually can be processed easily.

9.1.2.2 Branched Polymer

Branched polymer has the following chain structure (Fig. 9.2).

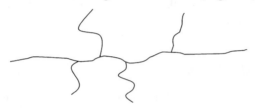

Figure 9.2 Branched polymer chain

Branched polymer has similar chemical properties to linear polymer. However, the physical properties of the branched polymer can be significantly affected by the formation of branch chains. For example, a linear polyethylene high density polyethylene (HDPE) has high crystallinity and density compared to branched low density polyethylene (LDPE) (Table 9.3).

Table 9.3 Crystallinity and Density of LDPE and HDPE

	General Structure	Crystallinity(%)	Density(g/cc)
LDPE	Linear with branching	50	0.92 – 0.94
HDPE	Linear with little branch	90	0.95

9.1.2.3 Crosslinked Polymer

Polymer chains can be linked together via chemical bonds to form a three dimensional network (Fig. 9.3). This type of polymer is called crosslinked polymer. Crosslinked polymer can neither be dissolved in solvents or be molten when heated. Crosslinked polymer is also called thermoset polymer.

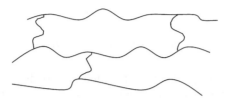

Figure 9.3 Crosslinked polymer chains (networks)

9.1.3 Polymer Thermal Behavior

Polymers can be classified as thermoplastic and thermoset polymers.

Thermoplastic — Both linear and branched polymers are thermoplastic.

Thermosetting — Crosslinked three dimensional, or network, polymers are thermoset polymers.

9.1.4 Polymer Stability

Polymeric materials can be divided into two main classes — biostable and bio-degradable polymers according to their stability when they are used in contact with biological systems.

Biodegradable polymer is a polymer in which the degradation is mediated at least partially by a biological system. The biodegradation of a polymer can be caused by hydrolytic, enzymatic or bacteriological degradation processes occurring within a polymer matrix. The degradation process will cause a deleterious change in the properties of a polymer due to a change in the chemical structure.

Most of the biodegradable polymers discovered so far contain hydrolysable linkages, such as ester and amide in their backbone structure. Among them, the flexible ester containing polymers, and in particular aliphatic polyesters, appear to be the most attractive biodegradable polymers because of their useful biodegradability and their versatility regarding physical, chemical and biological properties. Table 9.2 and Table 9.4 listed some examples of biostable and biodegradable polymers for biomedical applications.

Table 9.4 Some commonly seen synthetic biodegradable polymers

Polymer	Physical Characteristics	Applications
Poly(glycolic acid) (PGA)	Thermoplastic crystalline polymer $T_g^* = 225\,^\circ\text{C}$, $T_m^+ = 40\,^\circ\text{C} - 45\,^\circ\text{C}$	Absorbable suture and meshes

Continued

Polymer	Physical Characteristics	Applications
10/90 Poly (L-lactide-co-gly-colide)	Thermoplastic crystalline polymer $T_g = 43\,^{\circ}C$, $T_m = 205\,^{\circ}C$	Absorbable suture and meshes
Poly(p-dioxanone) (PDS)	Thermoplastic crystalline polymer $T_g = 10\,^{\circ}C$, $T_m = 110\,^{\circ}C - 115\,^{\circ}C$	Sutures
85/15 Poly (DL-lactide-co-glycoside)	Amorphous polymer $T_g = 50\,^{\circ}C - 55\,^{\circ}C$	Sutures
Poly(ε-caprolactone) (PCL)	Thermoplastic crystalline polymer $T_g = -60\,^{\circ}C$, $T_m = 59\,^{\circ}C - 64\,^{\circ}C$	Sutures

* T_g—glass transition temperature

\+ T_m—melting temperature

9.2 Characteristics of Polymer

Polymers have long chain structures that render the polymer unique physico-chemical properties when in comparison with other types of materials such as ceramic and metals. Many terms, some of them are unique to polymers, are used to describe polymer structure as well as the properties of polymer.

9.2.1 Degree of Polymerization

Each type of natural polymer, such as protein, usually has a specific molecular weight(MW), and is said to be monodisperse with respect to molecular weight. However, synthetic polymers, such as high density polyethylene (HDPE), are made up of molecules of different molecular weight.

$$\left[H_2C - CH_2 \right]_n$$

Thus, the numerical value for n (see the following formula), or the degree of polymerization (DP) should be considered as an average DP. Accordingly, the average molecular weight of a polydisperse polymer will equal the product of the average DP and the molecular weight of the repeat unit or mer

$$\overline{Mw} = (\overline{DP}) \times (M.\ W.\ \text{of mer})$$

147

9.2.2   Polymer Crystals

Polymer can form crystals. It is recognized that ordered polymers might form lamellar crystals with a thickness of $10 - 20$ nm in which the polymer chains are folded back on themselves to produce parallel chains perpendicular to the face of the crystals.

9.2.3   The Glass Transition Temperature and Melting Temperature

It is well known that temperature change will affect the physical properties of plastic. When the temperature increases, a plastic become soft, and then melt when the temperature increased further above a certain temperature. This temperature is usually called a melting temperature, or T_m. When the polymer T_m, those polymer crystals begin to fall apart or melt. The chains come out of their ordered arrangements, and begin to move around freely. As described above, melting is something that happens to a crystalline polymer.

Temperature also will affect the physical properties of amorphous regions. And there is a specific temperature associated with the effect. This temperature is called a glass transition temperature (T_g). When the polymer is cooled below this temperature, it becomes hard and brittle, like glass. Glass transition is a unique transition that only happens to polymers and not to other materials. Glass transition temperature is a very important temperature for amorphous polymers. For example, some polymers are used above their T_g, and some are used below T_g. When a polymer has a T_g higher than room temperature, then the polymer is in a glass state. So the polymer is a hard plastic. Examples are polystyrene and PMMA, two well known plastics at room temperature. Both of the two plastics have T_g around $100\,^{\circ}$C which is well above room temperature. When a polymer has a lower T_g well below the room temperature, the polymer behaves like a rubber. For example, elastomers like polyisoprene and polyisobutylene are soft and flexible when they used at room temperature which is above their T_g's.

It is important to note that glass transition is different from melting. Glass transition is a transition temperature happens to the amorphous region of polymers, while melting is a transition which occurs in crystalline region of polymers. When melting happens to the crystalline region of polymers, the ordered crystal structure is disrupted and the polymer chains start to move freely under the applied force of gravity.

As discussed early, even a crystalline polymer cannot have 100% crystallinity. Therefore, a crystalline polymer usually has an amorphous portion which coexists with the crystalline portion. This is why the same sample of a polymer can have both a glass transition temperature and a melting temperature. The T_m usually is higher than T_g because it takes much more energy to melt the crystal of polymers.

9.3   Synthesis of Polymers

9.3.1   Free Radical Polymerization

Free radical polymerization is one of the most common and useful reactions for preparation polymers. It is used to make polymers from vinyl monomers, that is, from small molecules containing carbon-carbon double bonds. Polymers made by free radical polymerization include commonly seen polystyrene, poly (methyl methacrylate), poly(vinyl chloride) and polyethylene. Free radical polymerization is a rapid reaction consists of 3 steps, namely, initiation, propagation and termination.

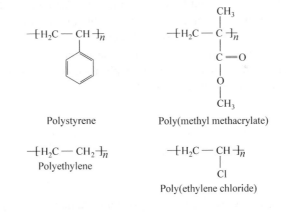

Polystyrene   Poly(methyl methacrylate)

Polyethylene   Poly(ethylene chloride)

Initiation

To start a radical polymerization, a molecule called an initiator is needed. Fig. 9.2 showed two typical initiators, 2, 2'-azo-*bis*-isobutyrylnitrile (AIBN) and benzoyl peroxide. Upon heating these initiators can generate initiator fragments that each of which has one unpaired electron (9.1), (9.2), (9.3). Molecules like this, with unpaired electrons are called free radicals.

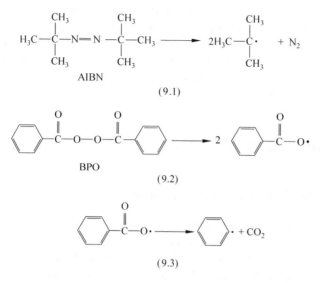

(9.1)

(9.2)

(9.3)

Propagation

The generated free radical then will react with monomers which have unsaturated bonds. The carbon-carbon double bond in a vinyl monomer, such as ethylene, is very easily attacked by the free radical. Then a new chemical bond between the initiator fragment and one of the double bond carbons of the monomer molecule will form and a new free radical species is produced at the same time. This whole process, the breakdown of the initiator molecule to form radicals, followed by the radical's reaction with a monomer molecule is called the initiation step of the polymerization (9.4).

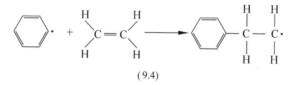

(9.4)

This newly formed free radical reacts with another ethylene molecule in the exact same way as the initiator fragment did. During the polymerization process, this reaction takes place over and over again and results in an increase in chain length.

This process, the adding of more and more monomer molecules to the growing chains, is called propagation.

Unless the newly formed radical is terminated and loss its reactivity, this propagation process will continue and a long chain will be formed (9.5). The reactions like this are called chain reactions.

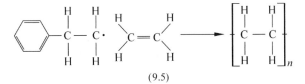

(9.5)

Termination

Radicals are extremely reactive and unstable. Not only the radicals will re-act with monomers, which result in an increase in chain length, but also the radicals can react with each other. When two radicals react with each other, there will be no new radical generated and the chain reaction will come to an end. This reaction is called termination reaction. Termination reaction happens in several ways. The simplest way is for two growing radical chains to react with each other as mentioned above. The two unpaired electrons from each radical chain then join to form a new chemical bond linking their respective chains. This is called coupling.

Coupling (9.6) is one of two main types of termination reaction.

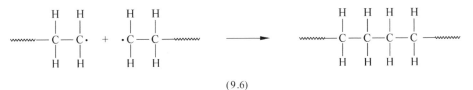

(9.6)

Another termination reaction is called disproportionation. In disproportiona-tion, when two growing chain ends come close together, the unpaired electron of one chain attracts not only one of the electrons from the carbon-hydrogen bond of the carbon atom next to the other carbon radical, but the hydrogen at-om as well. As a result, a double bond at the end of the polymer chain is crea-ted. (See (9.7), (9.8))

Sometimes, the unpaired electron at the end of a growing chain will pair itself with an electron from a carbon-hydrogen bond along the backbone of ano-ther polymer chain. This leaves an unpaired electron, which is nowhere near the propagating chain end. This electron cannot form a double bond the same way as the electron from the last example did, but it will react with a monomer molecule. This will start a new chain growing out of the middle of the first chain. This is called chain transfer to polymer, and the result is a branched polymer. This chain transfer could be a problem to some types of polymers when a linear chain structure is wanted, such as polyethylene. It is impossible

9.3 Synthesis of Polymers

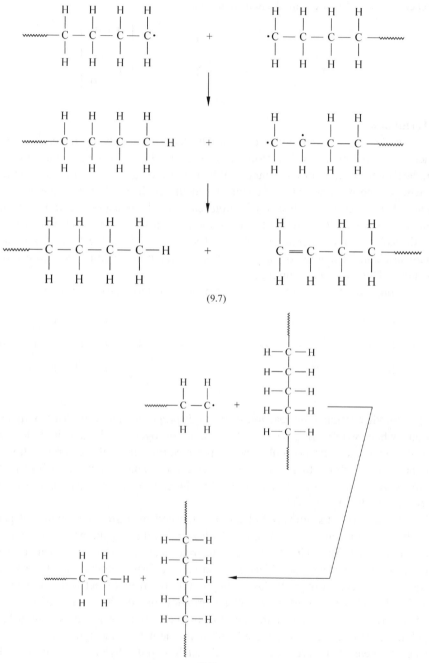

(9.7)

(9.8)

to get linear non-branched polyethylene by free radical polymerization. (See (9.9))

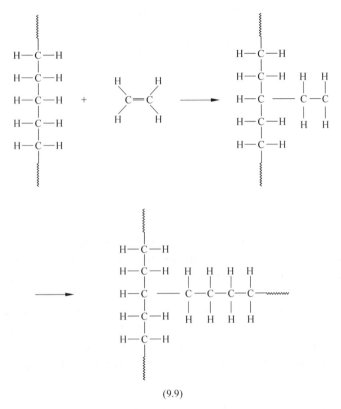

(9.9)

9.3.2 Condensation Polymerization

Another type of polymerization is called condensation polymerization. In an addition polymerization, the entire monomer molecule becomes part of the polymer. However, in a condensation polymerization, monomer molecules polymerizes into long chain polymers but also produce small molecules byproduct, such as water and HCl.

Condensation polymerization has a step growth kinetics, which means that the molecule weight of the polymer increases in a slow, step-like manner as reaction time increases. Following is an example (9.10) of making nylon 6,6 using adipoyl chloride and hexamethylene diamine. Aside from the product nylon 6, 6, a byproduct of HCl is also produced. Since the final polymer obtained has less mass than the original monomers, it is often said that the polymer is condensed with regard to the monomers.

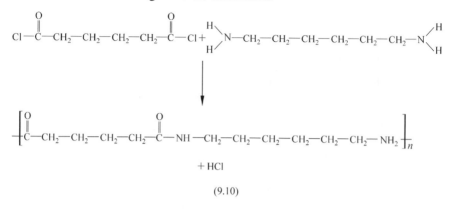

(9.10)

The polymerization proceeds by producing dimmer, trimer, tetramer, etc. in a step growth manner as the reaction progresses. This growth continues until some termination reaction happens. Therefore, this polymerization is also called stepwise polymerization.

It has to be noted that the condensation polymerization and stepwise polymerization are not the same. For example, the formation of polyurethanes and polyureas typically occurs through a stepwise polymerization. But no byproduct is released through the condensation of isocyanate with diol or diamine.

9.3.3 Other Types of Polymerization

9.3.3.1 Ionic Chain Reaction

Like free radical chain reaction, ionic chain reaction polymerization is fast. And the initiated species continue to propagate until termination. The initiator may be an anion or a cation. The polymerization also consists of three steps — initiation, propagation and termination, just like in a free radical polymerization.

Although most of the vinyl monomers undergo free radical polymerization, a small number of vinyl monomers undergo ionic polymerization. Cationic polymerization requires monomers that have electron-releasing groups such as an alkoxy, a phenyl, or a vinyl group. Anionic polymerization occurs with monomers containing electron-withdrawing groups, such as carboxyl, nitrile, or halide.

Comparing with free radical polymerization, ionic polymerizations can use heterogeneous initiators and they are usually quite sensitive to the presence of impurities, such as water. The selection of solvent for carrying out polymerization is very important as the ionic species formed during the polymerization are often not stable and can be destroyed by polar solvents such as water and alcohol. Therefore, ionic polymerizations are often carried out in low or moderate polar solvents, such as hexane and ethylene dichloride.

9.3.3.2 Complex Coordinative Polymerization

A catalyst called Ziegler-Natta catalyst is used in this type of polymerization. Ziegler-Natta catalyst is a combination of transition metal compound from Groups IV to VIII and an organometalic compound of a metal from groups I to III of the periodic table. However, the transition metal compound, such as $TiCl_4$, is generally referred to as the catalyst, and the organometalic compound, such as diethylaluminum chloride as cocatalyst.

For most of the vinyl monomers, use of Ziegler-Natta catalysts will produce polymers with isotactic form. The degree of steroregulation seems to be dependent on the amount of exposure of the active site.

9.3.3.3 Copolymerization

Copolymerization is not a polymerization mechanism, but rather a way to synthesis copolymers in order to get polymers with different properties than any of the homopolymers from their corresponding monomers. Copolymers can be synthesized by step reaction or by chain reaction (radical, ionic) polymerization.

Copolymers can be alternating copolymers, in which the monomer M_1 and M_2 are arranged in a regular alternating order in the chain.

$$—M_1M_2\ M_1M_2\ M_1M_2\ M_1M_2—$$

Random copolymers, in which the monomer sequences of M_1 and M_2 are arranged in a random fashion,

$$—M_1\ M_2\ M_1\ M_1M_2M_2M_1M_2—$$

Block copolymers, in which there are long sequences of the same repeating unit in the chain,

$$—(M_1)_m(M_2)_n—$$

Grafting polymer, in which the chain extension of the second monomer M_2 is as shown:

$$
\begin{array}{c}
| \\
M_1 \\
M_1 \\
M_1 \\
M_1 - (M_2)_n - \\
M_1 \\
M_1 \\
M_1 \\
|
\end{array}
$$

Copolymerization is an effective way to disrupt the crystallization behavior of the homopolymer. Comparing to the thermal behavior of homopolymers, copolymer can have a number of different transition temperatures depending on the type of copolymers (random, alternating, block, or grafting). For example, a random homopolymer can exhibit a T_g, which is approximately the weight average of the T_g's of the two homopolymers. Block and grafting copolymers can form two types of separate domains mainly consisting of segments of M_1 and M_2, respectively. Each type of domain, therefore, will exhibit a T_g close to these of each homopolymer.

Base on the above discussion, it is obvious that a copolymerization is a very useful method to modify the properties of homopolymers.

9.4　References

1. Ratner, B. D. Biomaterials science: an interdisciplinary endeavor. In: Biomaterials Science. In: B. D. Ratner, A. S. Hoffman, F. J. Schoen, J. E. lemons, eds. Academic Press, San Diego, p. 6 (1996)
2. Katz, J., Developments in medical polymers for biomaterials applications. Medical Device & Diagnostic Industry. Jan. p. 122 (2001)
3. Carraher C. E., Jr. Polymer Chemistry, 5th Ed. Marcel Dekker, Inc., New York, p. 165 – 229 (2000)
4. Odian, G., Principles of Polymerization, 3rd ed. Wiley-Interscience (1991)
5. http://www.psrc.usm.edu/macrog/index.htm

9.5 Problems

1. Determine the approximate number of repeat units (DP) for a polypropylene chain with a MW of 5.4×10^4.

2. If some head-to head configuration is detected in a polymer chain known to propagate by head-to-tail addition, what type of termination has occurred?

3. In general, which polymerization is more rapid: (a) free radical chain reaction or (b) step reaction polymerization?

4. If one obtained a yield of 10% polymer after 10 min of polymerization styrene by a free radical mechanism, what would be the composition of the other 90%?

5. Which of the following will yield a polymer when condensed with adipic acid: (a) ethanol, (b) ethylene glycol, (c) glycerol, (d) aniline, or (e) ethylenediamine?

6. What is the first product produced when a molecule of sebacyl chloride reacts with a molecule of ethylene glycol?

7. What would be the better or stronger fiber: one made from an ester of (a) terephthalic acid or (b) phthalic acid?

8. What is the most widely used catalyst for the production of HDPE.

9. What are the 4 different types of copolymers?

10. What is the difference between a thermoset polymer and a thermoplastic polymer? What is the difference in their chemical structure?

11. Chemically, what is the difference between glassy and rubbery polymers?

12. What is T_g?

10　Naturally Occurring Polymer Biomaterials

Naturally occurring polymers are used as biomaterials largely because their structures are similar to the human tissue they intend to replace. They are also available cheaply and easily in large quantities. Usually, the naturally occurring biomaterials can be degraded by naturally occurring enzymes and therefore they are biodegradable, which offers an additional advantage over the use of synthetic non-biodegradable polymers. However, the use of naturally occurring polymers often has the problem to provoke immune reaction of the host tissue. Therefore, many of the naturally occurring polymers have to be chemically modified before they are used as biomaterials.

10.1　General Introduction to Proteins

Proteins are monodisperse polymers of amino acids. They are essential components of plants and animals. There are twenty different α-amino acids, which can join together by peptide linkages to form polyamides or polypeptides. Polypeptides are often used by biologists to denote oligomers or relatively low molecular weight proteins. All α-amino acids found in proteins, except glycine (Gly), contain a chiral carbon atom and are L-amino acids.

Because amino acids have both amino and carboxylic groups, they can be ionized. The net ionic charge of an amino acid varies with changes of solution pH. At certain pH an amino acid can be electrically neutral and this pH is called isoelectric point. For simple amino acids which contain only one acid and one amine groups, this isoelectric point occurs at a pH about 6 at which a dipole or zwitterion is formed, as shown below.

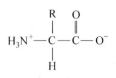

Because these amino acids can be ionized, they are water-soluble polar compounds, which migrate toward an electrode at pH values other than that of the isoelectric point in a process called electrophoresis.

Proteins and polypipetides are composed of many different types of amino acids. When writing out sequences for proteins and polypeptides common practies is to use a three-letter abbreviation of the individual amino acids to illustrate the structure of the protein, starting with the N terminus to the left of the protein and going to the $C - O$ terminus to the right. For example, a trimer with the following structure becomes Gly—Ala—Ser or GlyAlaSer or GAS.

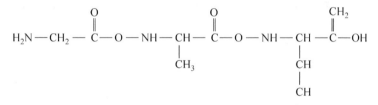

10.2   Collagen

Collagen, the most abundant protein in mammalian tissues, accounts for up to one-third of all protein mass in a mammal. Collagen fibers form the matrix or cement material in human bones where bone mineral precipitate. Collagen fibers constitute a major part of tendons and act as a major part of skin. The main function of collagen is the mechanical reinforcement of the connective tissues of vertebrates [1].

The individual polypeptide chains of collagen contain 20 different amino acids and the precise composition varies between different tissues. The variation in specific amino acid sequence gives rise to the different types of collagen labeled as Type I, Type II up to Type XIX. The most commonly occurring collagens are Types I, and III, which form the long-recognized characteristic fiber bundles seen in many tissues. Type I collagen is mostly found in skin, tendon, and bone, and Type III in blood vessels. The various collagen types show differences in degrees of glycosylation, which means that glucose and galactose are covalently coupled to the collagen molecules [2,3].

The lysine (Lys) and proline (Pro) residues present in the collagen are partly hydroxylated yielding the rare amino acids hydroxyproline (Hyp) and hydroxylysine (Hyl), respectively. Because the fiber forming collagen types are most abundant, their structure is discussed in more detail below.

The name collagen is used as a generic term to cover a wide range of protein molecules, which form supramolecular matrix structures. The basic building block of collagen is a triple helix of three polypeptide chains called the tropocollagen unit. Each chain is about 1,000 amino acid residues long. These three individual α-chains are cross-linked biosynthetically and fold to form a triple helix (tertiary structure) with a molecular weight of approximately 300.000 g/mol, a length of approximately 300 nm and a diameter of 1.5 nm [2, 3]. This triple-helix generates a symmetrical pattern of three left-handed helical α-chains (secondary structure), forming an additional "supercoil" with a pitch of 86 Å. The amino acids within each chain are displaced by a distance of 2.91 Å, with a relative twist of $-110°$, making the number of residues per turn 3.27 and the distance between each third glycine 8.7 Å[3] (See Fig. 10.1).

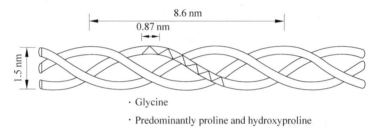

· Glycine

· Predominantly proline and hydroxyproline

Figure 10.1 Triple helix structure of collagen molecule

The presence of the cyclic imino acids, Pro and Hyp imparts rigidity and stability to the coil. Glycine (Gly), the smallest amino acid, must be in every third position in order to create the right-handed triple helix. Furthermore, the hydroxyl groups of Hyp residues are involved in hydrogen bonding and are important for stabilizing the triple-helix structure. Two hydrogen bonds per triplet are found. The two hydrogen bonds formed are: one between the NH-group of a glycyl residue with the CO-group of the residue in the second position of the triplet in the adjacent chain, and one via the water molecule participating in the formation of additional hydrogen bonds with the help of the hydroxyl group of Hyp in the third position. Such a ' water-bridged' model of the triple helix has been confirmed by physiochemical studies of the collagen molecule in solution and is supported by the observation that the thermal stability of the helix is dependent on the content of Hyp and not of Pro [4]. In addition, model studies showed that Gly, Hyp and Pro are the triple-helix forming amino acids and that only molecules which contain the triplets Gly-Pro-Hyp were able to form a helical structure. Therefore, the collagen triple helical domains have an amino acid sequence (primary structure) that is rich in Gly, Pro and Hyp.

The collagen molecules possess an axial periodicity that is visible in the electron microscope and pack into lattices with lateral symmetry (quaternary structure). This supramolecular structure is widely accepted as the microfibril containing five collagen triple-helices, with a diameter between 3.5 nm and 4.0 nm. Approximately 1,000 microfibrils can aggregate laterally and end-to-end into a fibril having a diameter of 80 − 100 nm, that displays a regular banding structure with a period of 65 nm (Fig. 10.2). About 500 fibrils form a

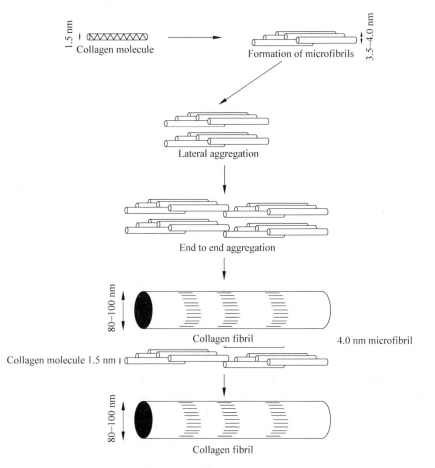

Figure 10. 2 Collagen fibril structure

collagen fiber with a diameter of 1 − 4 mm. Finally, the fibers aggregate into fiber bundles with a thickness between 10 and 100 mm. However, the hierarchy of the collagen is highly dependent on its function. For example, the fibril and fiber diameter of collagen in skin varies between 20 − 100 nm and 0. 3 − 40 mm, respectively. The diameter of the collagen fibril and fiber (fiber bundle) in tendons and ligaments is 20 − 250 nm and 1 − 300 mm, respectively. Collagen fibers are strong. In tendons, the collagen fibers have strength similar to that of hard-drawn copper wire [1].

Cross-linking makes these collagen stable and provide them with adequate tensile strength and visco-elasticity to perform their structural role. The cross-linking of collagen can take place naturally within the body through a reaction involves lysine side chains. Lysine side chains are oxidized to aldehydes that react with either a lysine residue or with one another through an aldol condensation and dehydration resulting in a cross-link. Intramolecular cross-links are formed by an aldol condensation reaction of two aldehyde groups. An intermolecular cross-link is formed if the aldehyde group reacts with the ε-amino group of an (hydroxy)lysine residue of an adjacent helix, yielding an aldimine or an Schiff base.

There has been an increased interest in the use of collagen and collagen-containing tissues in medical devices during the recent two decades. One way to use collagen-rich tissues is to chemically treat the tissue in order to make them into implantable prostheses. Examples are heart valves, vascular grafts, tendons, ligaments, and pericardium. Another way involves the use of purified collagen obtained from animal tissue, processed in a variety of ways to generate a large number of products that not only have applications in the medical field, but also in the manufacturing of cosmetics. Collagen can be used in the form of native soluble collagen, enzymatically processed native collagen, soluble collagen of reconstituted fibers, etc. Products are used as dermal implants, implantable drug delivery vehicles, sponges, tubes and suture.

10. 2. 1　Cross-Linking of Collagen

When collagen is implanted *in vivo*, it is subjected to degradation by collagenases: which is presented naturally in wound sites. Collagen also frequently elicits an immune response of the host if the collagen is from an animal source. Further treatment of the collagenous tissue, such as introducing cross-link to collagen materials, is necessary in order to control the degradation and masking the antigenic properties attributed to these materials.

Many methods have been used to creating new additional chemical bonds between the collagen molecules, which not only reinforce the tissue to produce a tough and strong but non-viable material, but also minimized the immogenicity of the collagen materials.

The obvious strategy would be the use of bifunctional reagents. Glutaraldehyde, epoxy and diisocyanate compounds were employed in this approach. Another strategy is to activate the carboxylic acid groups of collagen, followed by a reaction with an adjacent amine group. This method is the basis of using carbodiimide for collagen cross-linking reactions.

10.2.1.1   Glutaraldehyde

The predominant chemical agent that has been investigated for the treatment of collagenous tissues is glutaraldehyde, which gives materials the highest degree of cross-linking when compared with other known methods such as formaldehyde, epoxy compounds, cyanamide and the acyl-azide method. Glutaraldehyde was first applied successfully for heart valve bioprosthesis in the late 60s by Carpentier *et al.* Porcine aortic heart valves treated with glutaraldehyde showed good hemodynamic performance and a low antigenicity [7 –9].

The glutaraldehyde cross-linking reactions have been extensively studied. In general, it is believed that aldehydes react with the amine groups of (hydroxy)lysine residues of the collagen, yielding a Schiff base. However, the exact cross-linking structure is still not clear because a mixture of free aldehyde and mono- and dihydrated glutaraldehyde and monomeric and polymeric hemiacetals is always present in a glutaraldehyde aqueous solution.

The cross-linking reaction can be carried out using an aqueous glutaraldehyde solution at room temperature or even at $4°C$.

However, it is now known that the durability of glutaraldehyde fixed biological tissue is not so good as once thought before. In young patients who received glutaraldehyde cross-linked bioprosthetic heart valves the implanted heart valves can calcify severely, which is the major cause of the failure of bioprosthetic heart valves [9 –11]. Moreover, depolymerization of polymeric glutaraldehyde cross-links has been reported. This depolymerization releases monomeric glutaraldehyde which is highly cytotoxic to the recipient [12].

10.2.1.2   Epoxy Compounds

Bi- and trifunctional glycidyl ethers based on glycerol are used to cross-link collagen based materials including porcing aortic heart valves (see (10.1)) [13 –16]. In addition, a broad range of multifunctional epoxy containing cross-linkers can be used. Due to its highly strained three-membered ring, epoxide groups are susceptible to a nucleophilic attack. The cross-linking reaction mechanisim pH dependent. At a pH below 6, the cross-linking reaction involves the reaction between epoxide and carboxylic groups of aspartic and glutamic acid and results in the formation of ester bonds [17]. At a basic pH (pH >8), the reaction is predominantly a reaction of epoxide with the amine groups of (hydroxy)lysine residues as shown below (See(10.1)).

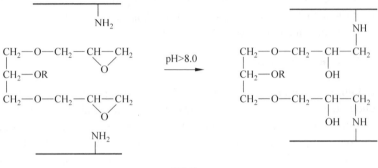

(10.1)

Additionally, epoxide groups react with the secondary amine groups of histidine. The fact that epoxy compound can react with both the carboxyle acid groups and amine groups increases the versatility of the cross-linking.

10.2.1.3 Carbodiimides

The carbodiimide reagent can induce cross-links between carboxylic acid and amine groups without itself being incorporated. The commonly used carbodiimide is a water-soluble carbodiimide called 1-ethyl-3-(3-dimethyl aminopropyl) carbodiimide (EDC) [17 – 19]. EDC cross-linking involves the activation of the carboxylic acid groups of Asp or Glu residues by EDC to give O-acylisourea groups. Besides EDC, another reagent N-hydroxysuccinimide (NHS) is used in the reaction for the purpose of suppressing side reactions of O-acylisourea groups such as hydrolysis and the N-acylshift. NHS can convert the O-acylisourea group into a NHS activated carboxylic acid group, which is very reactive towards amine groups of (hydroxy)lysine, yielding a so-called zero-length cross-link. In this cross-linking process, both EDC and NHS are not incorporated in the matrix (See(10.2)).

10.2.1.4 Other Bifunctional Cross-Linking Agents

Other bifunctional cross-linkers have been applied in the cross-linking of collagen such as hexamethylene diisocyanate [19], dimethyl suberimidate [20] and bis-N-hydroxysuccinimide ester derivates [21].

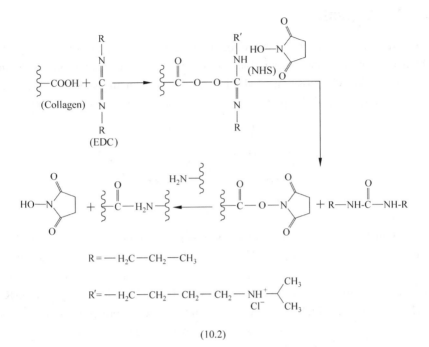

$$R = — H_2C—CH_2—CH_3$$

$$R' = — H_2C—CH_2—CH_2—CH_2—NH^+\!\!\!\overset{CH_3}{\underset{Cl^-\ \ CH_3}{<}}$$

(10.2)

10. 2. 1. 5   Physical Cross-Linking

The primary advantage of physical treatments is that they do not introduce chemicals that cause potential harm. Typical processes such as heating, drying and irradiation have been applied to collagen. Short wavelength ultraviolet (UV) irradiation (254 nm) can introduce cross-links in the collagen [22]. However, chain scission may become a substantial side reaction resulting in the denaturation of the collagen molecules.

Dehydrothermal treatment (DHT) promotes the condensation of carboxylic groups and amino groups in collagen by removing the aqueous products of condensation. This condensation reaction leads to the formation of inter-chain amide links. During DHT cross-linking, collagen is extensively dried in vacuum for several days at temperatures up to 110°C [23, 24]. Generally, the degree of cross-linking is considerably lower than obtained by chemical methods.

10.3 Alginate

Alginates are cell-wall constituents of brown algae (Phaeophycota). They are chain-forming heteropolysaccharides made up of blocks of mannuronic acid and guluronic acid. Composition of the blocks depends on the species being used for the extraction and the part of the thallus from which extraction is made.

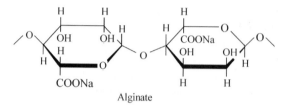

Alginate

Alginates are linear unbranched polymers containing β-(1→4)-linked D-mannuronic acid (M) and α-(1→4)-linked L-guluronic acid (G) residues. According to the source algae, alginates can consist of blocks of similar and strictly alternating residues (i. e. MMMMMM, GGGGGG and GMGMG-MGM), each of which have different conformational preferences and behavior. Alginates may be prepared with a wide range of average molecular weights (50 – 100,000 residues) to suit the application.

Because of their abundance in source and low in prices, Alginates have been widely used in the food and pharmaceutical industry as thickeners, emulsifying agents, binder and disintegrating agent for tablet and capsule formulations. Because of their biocompatibility, alginates have been used in medical applications such as wound dressings, scaffolds for tissue engineering and hepatocyte culture and surgical or dental impression materials [25 – 28]. Alginates are also known to be broken down to simpler glucose type residues and can be totally absorbed [26].

When used as biomaterials for implantation or tissue engineering scaffolds, alginates have to be cross-linked. Alginate can be easily cross-linked by calcium ions to form ionic bonding between alginate molecules. The cross-link is a fast process. As an example, cross-linked alginate beads can be obtained instantly by dripping sodium alginate solution into calcium chloride solution. Because of this useful characteristics, living cells, growth factors and other active ingredients can be easily encapsulated into calcium ion cross-linked alginate gels. The cross-linked alginate gel can act as an a immunoprotection barrier for its encapsulated living cells. Alginates cross-linked with calcium ions (from $CaSO_4$) have recently been used as cell delivery vehicles for *in vivo* tissue engineering research [29].

Alginate can also be easily fabricated into fibers. The fibers can be used to make non-woven fibers for medical applications. For example, non-woven calcium alginate fiber dressings have been used frequently on both full- and partial-thickness wounds. Many studies have shown that these alginate dressings can accelerate epithelialization [26, 30].

Alginate can also be covalently cross-linked using ethylenediamine in the presence of water-soluble carbodiimide, as carbodiimide will induce cross-links between carboxylic acid and amine groups without itself being incorporated. So ethylenediamine is actually being incorporated as a cross-linker. The covalently cross-linked membrane is easily biodegradable and can reduce foreign-body reactions after healing skin wounds [31].

10. 4   Chitin and Chitosan

Chitin is one of the most abundant polysaccharides found in nature. It is found naturally in the shells of crustaceans, insect exoskeletons, fungal cell walls, micro fauna and plankton. It is found in association with proteins and minerals such as Calcium Carbonate. Chitin is a homopolymer of 2-acetamido-2-deoxy-D-glucose (N-acetylglucosamine) $1 \rightarrow 4$ linked in a β configuration forming a long chain linear polymer. It is thus an amino sugar analog of cellulose [32]. Chitin is insoluble in most solvents.

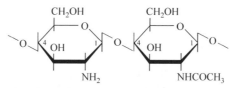

Chitosan is a useful derivative of chitin by removing most of the acetyl groups of chitin using strong alkalis. To obtain a soluble product the degree of deacetylation of chitosan must be 80% to 85% or higher; i. e. the acetyl content of the chitosan product must be less than $4\% -4.5\%$. Chitosan is a semi-crystalline polymer and the degree of crystallinity is a function of the degree of deacetylation [33].

Crystallinity is maximum for both chitin (i. e. 0% deacetylated) and fully deacetylated chitosan. Minimum crystallinity is achieved at intermediate degrees of deacetylation. Because of the stable, crystalline structure, chitosan is normally insoluble in both organic solvents and aqueous solutions at a pH above 7. However, it dissolves readily in most dilute organic acids solutions, such as formic, acetic, tartaric, and citric acids because the free amino groups are protonated and the molecule become fully soluble below pH 5. Chitosan is soluble to a limited extent in dilute inorganic acids except phosphoric and sulfuric acids. The pH-dependent solubility of chitosan is a very useful property, which provides a convenient mechanism for processing chitosan products under mild conditions. For example, viscous solutions of chitosan can be prepared at lower pH and then extruded and gelled in high pH solutions or baths of nonsolvents such as methanol. The obtained gel fibers can be subsequently drawn and dried to form high-strength fibers [34 – 36].

Depending on the source and preparation procedure, chitosan's average molecular weight may range from 50 to 1, 000 kDa. Commercially available preparations have degrees of deacetylation ranging from 50% to 90% [37].

Animal study showed that chitosan does not evoke any inflammatory or allergic reaction following implantation. Chitosan can be hydrolyzed by lysozyme. The degradation products of chitosan are amino sugars, which can be incorporated into glycosaminoglycan and glycoprotein metabolic pathways or excreted [38 – 40].

Chitosan also shows antimicrobial and antifungic activities [41] which makes it a favorable option for biomedical applications. It has been proven to be useful in promoting tissue growth in soft tissue repair, bone regeneration and cartilage regeneration [37, 41 – 43]. Moreover, chitosan can be incorporated into hydrogels and microspheres as delivery systems for drugs, proteins or genes [31].

10. 5   References

1. Carraher, C. E., Jr. Polymer Chemistry, 5th Ed. Marcel Dekker, New York (2000)
2. Zeeman, R., Crosslinking of collagen based materials. FEBODRUK BV., Enschede, The Netherlands (1998)
3. Nimni, M. E., R. D. Harkness. Molecular structure and functions of collagen. In: M. E. Nimni, ed. Collagen Volume I : Biochemistry, CRC Press, Inc., Boca Raton, Florida, USA (1988)
4. Weiss, J. B., S. Ayed. An introduction to collagen. In: J. B. Weiss, M. I. V. Jayson, eds. Collagen in health and disease, Churchill Livingstone, Edinburgh (1982)
5. Silver, F. H., G. D. Pins, M. -C. Wang, D. Christiansen. Collagenous biomaterials as models of tissue inducing implants. In: D. L. Wise, et al., eds. Encyclopedic handbook of biomaterials and bioengineering, Marcel Dekker, Inc., New York. pp. 1245 – 1266 (1995)
6. Sabelman, E. E., Biology, biotechnology, and biocompatibility of collagen. In: D. F. Williams, eds. Biocompatibility of tissue analogs, CRC Press Inc., Boca Raton (1985)
7. Jayakrishnan, A., S. R. Jameela. Glutaraldehyde as a fixative in bioprosthetic and drug

delivery matrices. Biomaterials **17**: 471 – 484 (1996)

8. Dunn, M. G., P. N. Avasarala, J. P. Zawadsky. Optimization of extruded collagen fibers for ACL reconstruction. J. Biomed. Mat. Res., **27**: 1545 – 1552 (1993)

9. Schoen, F. J., Cardiac valve prostheses: Review of clinical status and contemporary biomaterials issues. J. Biomed. Mat. Res. : Appl. Biomat, **21**(A1) : 91 – 117 (1987)

10. Nimni, M. E., D. Myers, D. Ertl, B. Han. Factors which affect the calcification of tissue-derived bioprostheses. J. Biomed. Mat. Res. **35**: 351 – 357 (1997)

11. Olde Damink, L. H. H., P. J. Dijkstra, M. J. A. v. Luyn, P. B. v. Wachem, P. Nieuwenhuis, J. Feijen. Glutaraldehyde as crosslinking agent for collagen based biomaterials. J. Mat. Sci. : Mat. in Med. **6**: 460 – 472 (1995)

12. Huang-Lee, L. L. H., D. T. Cheung, M. E. Nimni. Biochemical changes and cytotoxicity associated with the degradation of polymeric glutaraldehyde derived crosslinks. J. Biomed. Mat. Res., **24**: 1185 – 1201 (1990)

13. Tu, R., S. H. Shen, D. Lin, C. Hata, K. Thyagarajan, Y. Noishiki, R. C. Quijano. Fixation of bioprosthetic tissues with monofunctional and multifunctional poly epoxy compounds. J. Biomed. Mat. Res., **28**: 677 – 684 (1994)

14. Lee, J. M., C. A. Pereira, L. W. K. Kan. Effect of molecular structure of poly (glycidyl ether) reagents on crosslinking and mechanical properties of bovine pericardial xenograft materials. J. Biomed. Mat. Res., **28**: 981 – 992 (1994)

15. Tang, Z., Y. Yue. Crosslinkage of collagen by polyglycidyl ethers. ASAIO J. **41**: 72 – 78 (1995)

16. Sung, H. -W., H. -L. Hsu, C. -C. Shih, D. -S. Lin. Cross-linking characteristics of biological tissue fixed with monofunctional or multifunctional epoxy compounds. Biomaterials **17**: (14) 1405 – 1410 (1996)

17. Olde Damink, L. H. H., P. J. Dijkstra, M. J. A. v. Luyn, P. B. v. Wachem, P. Nieuwenhuis, and J. Feijen. Cross-linking of dermal sheep collagen using a water-soluble carbodiimide, Biomaterials. **17**(**8**) : 765 – 774 (1996)

18. Lee, J. M., H. L. Edwards, C. A. Pereira, and I. S. Samii. Cross-linking of tissue-derived biomaterials in 1-ethyl-3-(dimethylaminopropyl)-carbodiimide. J. Mat. Sci. : Mat. in Med. **7**(**9**) : 531 – 542 (1996)

19. Staros, J. V., N-hydroxysulfosuccinimide active esters: Bis (N-hydroxysulfosuccinimide) esters of two dicarboxylic acids are hydrophilic, membrane-impermeant, protein cross-linkers, Biochem. **22**: 3950 – 3955 (1982)

20. Olde Damink, L. H. H., P. J. Dijkstra, M. J. A. v. Luyn, P. B. v. Wachem, P. Nieuwenhuis, and J. Feijen. Crosslinking of dermal sheep collagen using hexamethylene diisocyanate. J. Mat. Sci. : Mat in Med. **6**(**7**) : 429 – 434 (1995)

21. Davies, G. E., and G. R. Stark. Use of dimethylsuberimidate, a crosslinking reagent, in studying the subunit structure of oligomeric proteins. Proc. Nat. Acad. Sci. **66**: 651 – 656 (1970)

22. Weadock, K., R. M. Olsen, and F. H. Silver. Evaluation of collagen crosslinking techniques. Biomat. Med. Dev. Art. Org. . **11**(**4**) : 293 – 318 (1983 – 1984)

23. Yannas, I. V., and A. V. Tobolsky. Cross-linking of gelatin by dehydration. Nature, **215**: 509 – 510 (1967)

24. Weadock, K. S., E. J. Miller, E. L. Keuffel, and M. G. Dunn. Effect of physical cross-linking methods on collagen-fiber durability in proteolytic solutions. J. Biomed. Mat. Res. **32**: 221 – 226 (1996)

10.5 References

25. Patel, H. A., Process for preparing the alginate-containing wound dressing. US Patent **5**: 470,576 (1993)
26. Gilchrist, T., A. M. Martin. Wound treatment with Sorbsan alginate wound dressing. Biomaterials **15**:317 −320(1994)
27. Cottrell, I. W., P. Kovacs. Alginates. In: R. L. Davidson, ed. Handbook of Water-Soluble Gums and Resins. New York, McGraw-Hill(1980)
28. McGinity, J. W., M. A. Pepka. Alginic Acid. In: AH Kibbe, ed. Handbook of Pharmaceutical Excipients, 3rd Ed. Pharmaceutical Press
29. Fragonasa, E., M. Valenteb, M. Pozzi-Mucellib, R. Toffaninc, R. Rizzoa, F. Silvestrid F. Vitturaa. Articular cartilage repair in rabbits by using suspensions of allogenic chondrocytes in alginate. Biomaterials, **21**(8): 795 −801 (2000)
30. Agren, M. S., Four alginate dressings in the treatment of partial thickness wounds: a comparative experimental study. Br J. Plast. Surg., **49**:129 −134 (1996)
31. Suzuki, Y., M. Tanihara, Y. Nishimura, K. Suzuki, Y. Yamawaki, H. Kudo, Y. Kakimaru, Y. Shimizu. In Vivo Evaluation of a Novel Alginate Dressing. J. Biomed. Mater. Res. (Appl. Biomater.) **48**: 522 −527(1999)
32. Carraher, C. E., Jr. Polymer Chemistry, 5th Ed. Marcel Dekker, New York, p. 179 (2000)
33. Peniston, Q. P, E. Johnson. Process for the Manufacture of Chitosan. US Patent No. **4**: 195,175 (1980)
34. S, Hirano, T. Midorikawa. Novel method for the preparation of N-acylchitosan fiber and N- acylchitosan cellulose fiber. Biomaterials **19**(1 −3):293 −297 (1998)
35. Qin, Y, Agboh O. C. Chitin and chitosan fibres. Med. Dev. Technol. **9**(10):24 −28 (1998)
36. Rathke, T. D., S. M. Hudson. Review of chitin and chitosan as fiber and film formers. Rev. Macromol. Chem. Phys., **C34**:375 −437 (1994)
37. Suh, J.-K. F., H. W. T. Matthew. Application of chitosan-based polysaccharide biomaterials in cartilage tissue engineering: a review. Biomaterials **21**: 2589 − 2598 (2000)
38. Domard, A., M. Rinaudo. Preparation and characterization of fully deacetylated chitosan. Int. J. Biol. Macromol. **5**:49 −52 (1983)
39. Muzzarelli, R. A. A., Chitin and the human body. In First International Conference of the European Chitin Society. Advances in Chitin Science. Brest, pp. 448 −461 (1995)
40. Hirano, S., H. Tsuchida, N. Nagao. N-acetylation in chitosan and the rate of its enzymic hydrolysis. Biomaterials **10**(8):574 −576 (1989)
41. Dinesh, K. S., A. R. Ray. Biomedical application of chitin, chitosan, and their derivatives. J. Macromol. Sci. Chem. Phys. **C40**:69 −83 (2000)
42. Pianigiani, E., A. Andreassi, P. Taddeucci, C. Alessandrini, M. Fimiani, L. A. Andreassi. New model for studying differentiation and growth of epidermal cultures on hyaluronan-based carrier. Biomaterials **20**: 1689 −1694 (1999)
43. Mao, J., L Zhao, K. Yao, Q. Shang, G. Yang, Y. Cao. Study of novel chitosan-gelatin artificial skin in vitro. J. Biomed Mater. Res. **64A**: 301 −308 (2003)

10. 6 Problems

1. What are the advantages of using naturally occurring polymers as biomaterials?
2. Define a protein in polymer science language.
3. To which pole will an amino acid migrate at a pH above its isoelectric point?
4. Why is collagen stronger than albumin?
5. Why collagen has to be cross-linked before its use as an implant?
6. How to cross-link collagen without incorporating of cross-linking agent to its structure?
7. Why would you expect chitin to be soluble in hydrochloric acid?
8. Can you think of a way to cross-link chitosan?
9. Besides using calcium ions to cross-link alginate, can you think of another way to cross-link alginate?
10. How can you control the degradation rate of chitosan *in vivo*?

11 Synthetic Non-Biodegradable Polymers

Synthetic polymers have been widely used in making various medical devices, such as disposable supplies, implants, drug delivery systems and tissue engineering scaffolds. The advantages of using polymers, as biomaterials, are their manufacturability. Polymers are easy to fabricate into various sizes and shapes compared to metals and ceramics. They are also light in weight and with a wide range of mechanical properties for different applications.

Most commonly use non-biodegradable polymeric biomaterials are originally developed for non-biomedical use. Therefore, it is not surprising to know that there is a lot of drawbacks associated with these polymer biomaterials. However, there are still no newly engineered polymers that can replace these "old" biomaterials. They are still widely used nowadays, as reviewed below.

11. 1 Polyethylene

There are three type of polyethylene: linear high density polyethylene (HDPE), branched low density polyethylene (LDPE) and ultrahigh molecular weight polyethylene (UHMWPE). HDPE and UHMWPE are frequently used as biomaterials.

Table 11. 1 Typical average physical properties of high density polyethylene (HDPE), Ultra-High Molecular Weight Polyethylene (UHMWPE), adapted from [1]

Property	HDPE	UHMWPE
Molecular weight (106 g/mol)	0. 05 − 0. 25	2 − 6
Melting temperature (°C)	130 − 137	125 − 138
Poisson's ratio	0. 40	0. 46
Specific gravity	0. 952 − 0. 965	0. 932 − 0. 945
Tensile modulus of elasticity* (GPa)	0. 4 − 4. 0	0. 8 − 1. 6
Tensile yield strength* (MPa)	26 − 33	21 − 28
Tensile ultimate strength* (MPa)	22 − 31	39 − 48

| | | Continued |
Property	HDPE	UHMWPE
Tensile ultimate elongation* (%)	10 – 1,200	350 – 525
Impact strength, izod* (J/m of notch; 3. 175 mm thick specimen)	21 – 214	>1,070 (No Break)
Degree of crystallinity (%)	60 – 80	39 – 75

* Testing conducted at 23°C.

11.1.1   High Density Polyethylene

High density polyethylene(HDPE) is a very inert material with very low tissue reactivity. It has been used as bone and cartilage substitutes since 1940s. More than 30 years of follow-up results showed favorable response to these HDPE implants. Therefore, HDPE has become a standard reference material for bio-compatibility testing. Histological examination of HD implants reveals a lack of capsule formation and minimal inflammatory and foreign body reactions.

When HDPE was fabricated into porous scaffolds, it has the added advantages of allowing fibrous tissue ingrowth into the implant. The ingrowth of the fibrous tissue will provide adequate stabilization in a non-load-bearing environment. MedPor (Porex Surgical Inc.) is a porous HDPE product fabricated by sintering HDPE microbeads in a mold to create implants with interconnected porous structure. The average pore size in this material is greater than 100 μm and the pore volume is in the 50% range. This material is flexible at room temperature. When heated in hot water, it becomes malleable. These materials are readily available in a variety of preformed shapes and can be customized with a scalpel easily [2 – 4].

The pore size and porosity is very important for tissue ingrowth. Studies have shown that pore size larger than 100 μm encourages tissue ingrowth. The tissue ingrowth results in firm attachment and integration of the implant to the surrounding tissue leading to decreased migration of the implant, thus obviating the need for screw or suture fixation in some cases. The vascularized soft tissue network throughout the implants reduces the likelihood of infection. The rapidity of vascularizd tissue ingrowth in HDPE has been shown to make this material more resistant to infection than other porous implant materials. The degree of vacularization is such that implants modified *in situ* produced bleeding when cut with a scalpel.

Porous HDPE has been successfully used for craniofacial applications, such as chin, malar area, nasal reconstruction, ear reconstruction, orbital reconstruction, and the correction of craniofacial contour deformities [2 – 4].

11.1.2 Ultrahigh Molecular Weight Polyethylene

The ultrahigh molecular weight polyethylene (UHMWPE) powders have been produced using the Ziegler process by Ruhrchemie (currently known as Ticona) since the 1950s [5]. The main ingredients for producing UHMWPE are ethylene (an reactive gas), hydrogen and titanium tetra chloride (the catalyst). The polymerization takes place in a solvent used for mass and heat transfer.

UHMWPE is produced as powder and must be consolidated under elevated temperatures and pressures because of its high melt viscosity—the result of ultra high molecular weight. As already discussed previously, as the molecular weight increase, the molecular chain of PE start to entangle each other, so UHMWPE does not flow like lower molecular weight polyethylene when raised above its melting temperature. For this reason, many thermoplastic processing techniques, such as injection molding, screw extrusion, or blow molding, cannot be used for UHMWPE fabrication. Therefore, compression molding is a common method to produce finished or semi-finished UHMWPE.

UHMWPE powder can be converted to sheets, rods or other preformed shapes by compression molding to facilitate subsequent machining operations by orthopedic manufacturers. Due to the relatively low thermal conductivity of UHMWPE, the duration of the molding cycle will depend upon the particular geometry of the press and the size of the sheet to be produced, but the processing time can last up to 24 h. The long molding times are necessary to maintain the slow, uniform heating and cooling rates throughout the entire sheet during the molding process.

UHMWPE particles can also be converted to finished or semi-finished parts using individual molds. The advantage of direct molding is the extremely smooth surface finish obtained with a complete absence of machining marks at the articulating surface. Direct compression molding has been used for over twenty years to produce tibial and acetabular inserts.

UHMWPE possesses many attractive properties, notably high abrasion resistance, low friction, high impact strength, excellent toughness, low density, ease of fabrication, biocompatibility, and biostability. These properties make it very attractive for use in fabricating bearing surfaces in arthroplasties. In fact, UHMWPE is the sole material currently used for the manufacture of the liner of the aceabular cup in total hip arthroplasties (THAs) and the tibial insert and patellar component in total knee arthroplasties. In these cases, the clinical performance of the components is considered to be very good except for the concern about there wear [6, 7].

Hip replacement is one of the world's most common operations, with approximately half a million diseased or damaged joints replaced annually worldwide. The number of procedures is growing with a commensurate increase in revisions. After a number of failed attempts with fluorocarbons, success was achieved in the early 1960s in the production of total joint replacements (TJRs) with UHMWPE. This remains the preferred material because of its exceptional mechanical properties, chemical inertness, impact resistance, and low coefficient of friction.

The problem asociated with the use of UHMWPE is the wear debris that will evoke a series of undesirable effects. It has been hypothesized that these particles are phagocytosed, resulting in many "reactions": formation of grannulamatous lesions, osteolysis, and bone resorption.

11.2 Poly(methyl methacrylate)

Poly(methyl methacrylate) (PMMA) can be prepared by heat initiating the polymerization of methyl methacrylate (MMA) using initiators such as AIBN and BPO as described in Chapter 2. Chemists also discovered that MMA could be polymerized at room temperature in the presence of BPO and a co-initiator such as tertiary aromatic amines. In 1943, a protocol for the chemical production of bone cement was established in the companies of Degussa and Kulzer [8]. A lot of research and development work has been done since then. In 1958, Sir John Charnley first succeeded in anchoring femoral head prosthesis in the femur with two-part self-polymerizing PMMA. Since then, the PMMA bone cement (now known simply as bone cement) emerged as one of the premier synthetic biomaterials in contemporary orthopedics. It is currently the only material used for anchoring cemented arthroplasties to the contiguous bones [9].

A typical PMMA bone cement consists of two parts, a solid part in a packet and a liquid part in a vial (See Table 11.2). When the two parts are mixed before use, the viscosity of mixture will gradually increase and become the dough in a few minutes. The dough will harden in another few minutes. This process actually involves a MMA polymerization process. Polymer PMMA is used to minimize the shrinkage and the heat release caused by the polymerization of monomer MMA, because the pure MMA will exhibit a shrinkage of about 21% due to the change of density and the heat release which can cause the temperature to increase to over $100^{\circ}C$ [1, 2].

11.2 Poly(methyl methacrylate)

Table 11.2 Components of PMMA bone cement

Powder Packet	Liquid Vial
Packet of powder containing PMMA beads, 10% radiopaque barium sulphate (or sometimes zirconium dioxide), a polymerization initiator (1% of benzoyl peroxide)	Vial of liquid containing MMA monomer and an activator (about 3% of DMP toluidine) that promotes the cold curing process. Also a trace of polymerization inhibitor, such as hydroquinone, to minimize monomer polymerization during storage

Heat stable antibiotics, such as gentamycin, tobramycin, erythromycin, vancomycin, cephalosporin, can be added in a powder form to the powder part. Antibiotics can be slowly release to eliminate possible infections of the surgery (See (11.1)).

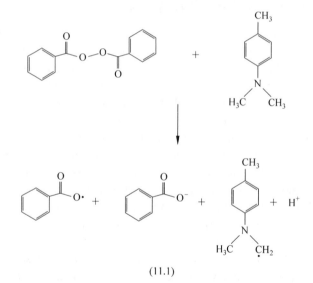

(11.1)

In most of the commercial bone cements, BPO and DMPT are used as initiator system. When the powder part is mixed with the liquid part, i.e. the BPO meets DMPT, free radicals will be produced at room temperature and thus the polymerization of MMA will be initiated. The polymerisation will result in the formation of long-chain polymers that are essentially linear and relatively free of crosslinking.

The curing process may be characterised by the following time periods:

(1) Dough time starts from the beginning of mixing and ends at the point when the bone cement mixture will not stick to unpowdered surgical gloves. This occurs approximately 2 to 3 min after the beginning of mixing for most PMMA cements. The ASTM specification for acrylic bone cement (ASTM F451-99a) specifies that the maxim dough time is 5.0 min. During this period, the monomer MMA wets and swells the PMMA beads. At the same time, the polymerisation is initiated. As the polymerisation goes on and the swelling of the PMMA beads, the viscosity of the cement systems increases and the cement behaves like a sticky dough.

(2) Working time is the time from the end of dough time until the cement is too stiff to manipulate, usually 5 – 8 min. During this period of time, the chain propagation continues and the viscosity of cement continues to increase until the cement becomes hardened. Cement can become very hot because the polymerisation process is an exothermic chemical reaction that liberates 12 – 14 kcal/100 g of typical bone cement.

(3) Setting time is the period measured from the beginning of mixture until the surface temperature of the dough mass is one-half its maximum value. It is the sum of the dough time and the working time. This is typically 8 – 10 min. According to ASTM F451-99a, the working time should be in the range of 5 – 15 min (See Fig. 11.1).

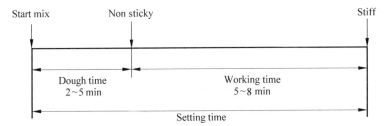

Figure 11.1 PMMA bone cement curing process

11.3 Polyester

Polyester is a family of polymers which have ester linkage connecting the polymers [10, 11].

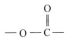

Among the polyester family, poly(ethylene terephthalate) (PET) is the world leading synthetic fibers and films. The typical synthetic reaction of PET uses dimethyl terephathalate and ethylene glycol (See (11.2)):

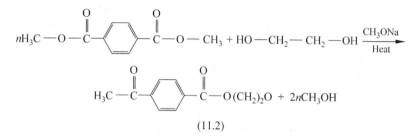

$$(11.2)$$

The synthesis of PET is a two-step process. First, dimethyl terephthalate is heated with ethylene glycol to obtain low molecular weight oligomers of PET. Then the mixture is heated to a higher temperature of 250 ℃ under vacuum to further promote the condensation reaction. The byproduct methanol is removed using vacuum and heat.

PET is considered to be biocompatible. It has very good mechanical properties. Therefore, PET fibers and the structures made from fibers, such as woven, knitted, felted and braided structures, are used as sutures (Mersilene[TM] and Ethibon[TM]), internal patches, pledgets, ligamentous prosthesis, artificial blood vessels, heart valve sewing cuffs, etc. [12].

11.4　Polycarbonate

Polycarbonate family polymers have carbonate linkages in their polymer chains [10, 11].

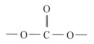

Polycarbonate can be synthesized by the reaction of phosgene with bisphenol A [2, 2-bis(4-hydroxyphenyl) propane]. The obtained PC is a tough and transparent plastic commercially available (See (11.3)).

Polycarbonate (e.g. Makrolon[TM] 2558) is used to make components for oxygenator for open heart surgery, venous reservoir, and arterial filter due to its sterilizability, ease of processing, biocompatibility, and clarity.

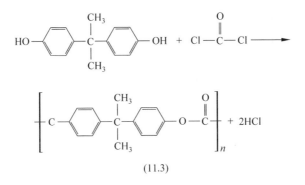

(11.3)

11.5 Polyamides

Polyamide polymers (nylon) have amide linkages in their polymer chains [10, 11].

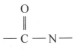

The first polyamide synthesized was Nylon-66. It was synthesized through the polycondensation of hexamethylenediamine and adipic acid (See (11.4)).

$$n\,HO-\overset{O}{\overset{\|}{C}}-(CH_2)_4-\overset{O}{\overset{\|}{C}}-OH \;+\; n\,H_2N-(CH_2)_6-NH_2 \xrightarrow{\text{Heat}}$$

$$\left[\overset{O}{\overset{\|}{C}}-(CH_2)_4-\overset{O}{\overset{\|}{C}}-O-NH-(CH_2)_6-NH\right]_n + 2n\,H_2O$$

(11.4)

By changing the dicarboxylic acid and diamine, different types of nylons can be prepared. The general structure of nylon (e. g. Nylon-*ab*) can be written, where *a* and *b* are equal to the number of carbon atoms in the repeating units of the diamine and dicarboxylic acid. For example, Nylon-610 and Nylon-612 are produced by the condensation of hexamethylenediamine and sebacic or dodecanoic acid, respectively. Nylon-6 is produced by the ring-opening polymerization of caprolactam.

Nylon has been used as surgical sutures. Sutures such as Ethilon™ and Nurolon™ are made from Nylon-6 or Nylon-66.

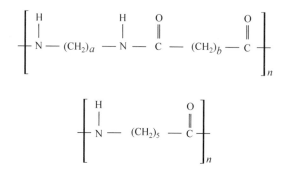

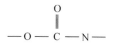

11.6 Polyurethane

Polyurethanes are a class of polymer with urethane linkage [10, 11]:

$$-O-\overset{\overset{\displaystyle O}{\|}}{C}-N-$$

Typically, polyurethane is synthesized by the reaction of dihydric alcohols and diisocyanates. For example, a crystalline polymer can be prepared by the reaction of 1,4-butanediol and hexamethylene diisocyanate as shown below (See (11.5)).

$$HO(CH_2)_4OH + nOCN(CH_2)_6NCO \longrightarrow$$

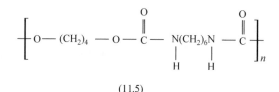

(11.5)

Diisocyanate with an even number of carbon atoms will produce higher melting polymers than those with an odd number of carbon atoms. The melting point is decreased as the number of methylene groups is increased, and increased by the incorporation of stiffening groups such as phenylene groups [10].

Polyurethane elastomers are frequently used as biomaterials due to their excellent fatigue resistant properties and biocompatibility. Polyurethane elastomers are segmented block copolymers containing so-called hard and soft segments (See(11.6)). The hard segments aggregate in domains held together by hydrogen bonding between the urethane segments. Therefore, the hard segment acts as a physical cross-linking point. The soft segments used in polyurethane elastomers are dihydroxy terminated long chain macroglycols with low T_gs. They include polyethers, polyesters, polydienes or polyolefins, and polydimethylsiloxanes (See (11.6)).

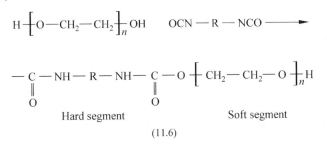

Hard segment Soft segment

(11.6)

Polyurethanes for biomedical uses are often synthesized via a two-step reaction process as illustrated in (11.7) [13]. In this method, the first step is to synthesis the prepolymer by reaction of the polyol with excess diisocyanate to form a diisocyanate terminated intermediate oligomer or a prepolymer. The second step is to convert this prepolymer to the final high molecular weight

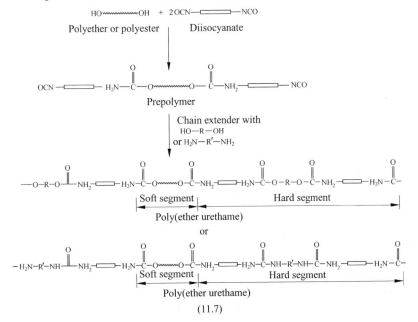

(11.7)

polyurethane by further reaction with a low Mw diol or diamine chain extender. This step is usually referred to as chain-extension.

It has to be noted that if a diamine chain extender is used, a urea linkage will be formed and this type of polyurethane is generally referred to as poly (ether urea urethane) (PEUU).

Polyurethane elastomers have traditionally been made from polyether or polyester soft segments. The diisocyanate commonly used are 2,4-toluene diisocyanate (TDI) and methylene di(4-phenyl isocyanate) (MDI). Polyester-based urethanes have relatively good material properties, but their ester linkages are susceptible to hydrolytic cleavage. Polyether-based urethanes have relatively high resistance to hydrolytic chain scission. Polyethylene oxide (PEO)-based urethanes exhibit poor water resistance due to the hydrophilic nature of the ethylene oxide. Polypropylene oxide (PPO) has been also widely used because of its low cost and reasonable hydrolytic stability, although the mechanical properties of urethanes made from polypropylene oxide are not as good as those made from polytetramethylene oxide (PTMO) or polyester [14].

Among the polyether-based polyurethane elastomers, the one made from the soft segment PTMO exhibits the best mechanical properties which are comparable to those of poly(ester urethanes). In addition, these polyurethanes show outstanding hydrolytic stability, good low temperature flexibility, good thermal stability, high fungus resistance, and an excellent abrasion resistance.

Low molecular weight diol and diamine chain extenders play a very important role in polyurethanes. Without a chain extender, a polyurethane formed by directly reacting diisocyanate and polyol generally has very poor physical properties and often does not exhibit microphase separation. Thus, the introduction of a chain extender can increase the hard segment length to permit hard-segment segregation, which results in excellent mechanical properties, such as an increase in the modulus and an increase in the hard-segment glass transition temperature (T_g) of the polymer. By changing the ratio of polyol to chain extender, polyurethanes can change from a hard, brittle thermoplastic to a rubbery elastomer [13, 14].

The biodegradation of polyurethane has been extensively studied. It has been found that several factors, such as chemical agents, stress, metal ions, physiological fluids, cells and enzymes are closely related to the polyurethane degradation *in vivo* [15−17].

Polyester urethanes are generally hydrolytically unstable when implanted in the human body, and therefore, their use is limited. Poly(ester urethanes) have been used as catheters and gastric balloons which only need to be used for a short period of time. These poly(ester-urethanes) are especially unstable in acidic environments. The acid-catalyzed hydrolysis of the ester linkage promotes further degradation of the poly(ester urethanes) by cleaving the urethane linkage. On the other hand, poly(ether urethanes) are hydrolytically stable. But they undergo *in vivo* degradation via different mechanisms, such as auto-oxidation, metal ion oxidation and environmental stress cracking [15 – 17].

In the metal ion oxidation degradation mechanism, it is believed that the degradation of the poly(ether urethane) is caused by the oxidation of the polyether soft segment. The oxidation of the polyether is catalyzed by the metal ions which are chelated by the polyether segments [18].

Environmental stress cracking of the poly(ether urethane) involves biological and physicochemical factors. The erosion of the poly(ether urethane) in such case started from the surface of the polymer, then propagated to the bulk, leading to the failure of the implanted device. It has been found again that the polyether segment is the target of this degradation. In this degradation mechanism, the inflammatory cells played a key role. Once these cells are activated, they release oxidative chemicals which oxidize the polyether bonds in poly (ether urethanes) [19].

It is clear that the polyether segments are the weak linkages of poly(ether urethane). Therefore, many researchers have been working on the synthesis of new polyurethanes by reducing the ether linkages in the soft segments or completely removing ether linkages from the soft segments.

Modifications or substitutions of the soft segment have been made to enhance biostability. The soft segment chemistries have been varied by substituting the polyether segment with a polybutadiene, polydimethylsiloxane (PDMS), polycarbonate, and aliphatic hydrocarbon segment. It has been shown that the polycarbonate soft segment is less likely to be cleaved via oxidation although hydrolysis of the carbonate linkage is possible. Results from many studies have confirmed that the polycarbonate soft segment is more stable than the polyether soft segment [20, 21]. Incorporation of PDMS as the soft segment into polyurethanes will rend the polyurethanes very attractive PDMS properties, such as good blood compatibility, low toxicity, good thermal and oxidative stability, low modulus, and anti-adhesive nature [22, 23].

Because of their excellent mechanical properties and biocompatibility, segmented polyurethanes have been frequently used in the medical devices in the past two decades as blood contacting materials, such as totally implantable artificial hearts and left ventricular assist devices (VADs). Poly(ether urethanes) were introduced as pacemaker lead insulators due to their hydrolytic stability.

11.7 Polysulfones

Polysulfons are a family of polymers which have linkages in their backbones [10, 11].

$$-\overset{\overset{\displaystyle O}{\|}}{\underset{\underset{\displaystyle O}{\|}}{S}}-$$

Polysulfones have excellent mechanical properties and chemical resistance. One of the important polysulfones is poly(aryl sulfones) which is synthesized by the following reaction (See (11.8)).

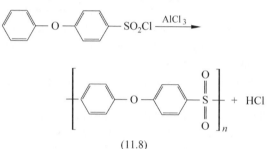

(11.8)

Some of the characteristics of polysulfones are:
(1) Heat resistant: Heat deflection temperature (HDT) 174°C;
(2) Excellent hydrolytic stability to hot water and steam sterilization;
(3) Excellent chemical resistance to inorganic acids & bases;
(4) Food, water and medical contact compliance.

They are used as membranes for hemodialysis. Polysulfones have been used as orthopeadic biomaterials due to their excellent mechanical properties (tensile modulus ~ 2.4 GPa). To improve their bone-bonding properties, polysulfones were used to make composites with bioactive glass.

11.8 Poly(ether ether ketone)

The structure of Poly(ether ether ketone) (PEEK) is

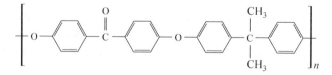

PEEK is a crystalline polymer with a glass transition temperature of 145 °C The most common form of PEEK is the one shown, derived from Bisphenol A, although limitless variations are possible, and a few are commercially produced. PEEK is a remarkable material, highly crystalline, thermally stable, resistant to many chemicals, and very tough. It can be melt-processed at very high temperatures (>300 °C), and is useful for special applications like pipes in oil refineries and chemical plants, and parts for scientific instruments, aerospace and biomedical devices where high price is not a limitation.

11.9   References

1. Edidin, A. A., S. M. Kurtz. The influence of mechanical behavior on the wear of four clinically relevant polymeric biomaterials in a hip simulator. J. Arthroplasty **15**: 321 – 331(2000)
2. Klawitter, J. J., J. G. Bagwell, A. M. Weinstein, BW Sauer. An evaluation of bone growth into porous high density polyethylene. J. Biomed. Mater. Res. **10**(2): 311 – 323 (1976)
3. Frodel, J. L., S. Lee. The use of high-density polyethylene implants in facial deformities. Arch. Otolaryngol Head Neck Surg. **124**(11): 1219-1223 (1998)
4. Wellisz, T., G. Kanel, R. V. Anooshian. Characteristics of the tissue response to MedPor porous polyethylene implants in the human facial skeleton. J. Long-term Effects Med. Implants. **3**: 223 – 235 (1993)
5. Birnkraut, H. W., Synthesis of UHMWPE. In: Ultra-High Molecular Weight Polyethylene as a Biomaterial in Orthopedic Surgery. Hogrefe & Huber Publishers (1991)
6. Lewis, G. Polyethylene wear in total hip and knee arthroplasties. J. Biomed. Mater. Res. (Appl. Biomater.) **38**: 55 – 75 (1997)
7. Li, S., A. H. Burstein. Ultra-high molecular weight polyethylene. The material and its use in total joint implants. J. Bone Joint Surg. Am. **76**: 1080 – 1090 (1994)
8. K-D Kühn. Bone Cements, Springer-Verlag (2002)
9. Lewis, G. Properties of acrylic bone cement: state of the art review. J. Biomed. Mater. Res. (Appl Biomater.) **38**: 155 – 182 (1997)
10. Carraher, C. E., Jr. Polymer Chemistry, 5th Ed, Marcel Dekker, Inc., New York (2000)
11. Odian, G. Principles of Polymerization. 3rd ed. Wiley-Interscience (1991)
12. King, M. W., Z. Zhang, R. Guidoin. Microstructure changes in polyester biotextiles during implantation in humans. J. Textile Apparel. Tech. & Management **1**(3): 1 – 8 (2001)
13. Lelah, M. D., S. L. Cooper. Polyurethane in Medicine. CRC Press, Boca Raton (1986)
14. Hepburn, C., Polyurethane Elastomer, 2nd. Ed. Elsevier Applied Science, New York (1992)
15. Griesser, H. J., Degradation of polyurethanes in biomedical applications — A review. Polymer Degradation and Stability **33**: 329 – 354 (1991)

16. Pinchuk, L., A review of the biostability and carcinogenicity of polyurethanes in medicine and the new generation of "biostable polyurethanes". J. Biomater. Sci. Polym. Edn. **6**: 225 – 267 (1994)

17. Stokes, K., R. McVenes, J. M. Anderson. Polyurethane elastomer biostability. J. Biomater. Appl. **9**: 321 – 354 (1995)

18. Stokes, K., A. J. Coury, P. Urbanski. Autooxidative degradation of implanted polyether polyurethane devices. J. Biomater. Appl. **1**: 411 – 448 (1987)

19. Zhao, Q., M. P. Agger M. Fitzpatrick, J. M. Anderson, A. Hiltner, K. Stokes, P. Urbanski. Cellular interaction with biomaterials: in vivo cracking of pre-stressed Pellethane 2363-80A. J. Biomed. Mater. Res. **24**: 621 – 637 (1990)

20. Phaneuf, M. D., W. C. Quist, F. W. Logerfo, M. Szycher, D. J. Dempsey, M. J. Bide. Chemical and physical characterization of a novel poly(carbonate urea) urethane surface with protein crosslinker sites. J. Biomaterials Appl. **12**: 100 – 120 (1997)

21. Tanzi, M. C., S. Fare, Paola Petrini. In vitro stability of polyether and polycarbonate urethanes). J. Biomaterials Appl. **14**: 325 – 348 (2000)

22. Park, J. H., K. D. Park, Y. H. Bae. PDMS-based polyurethanes with MPEG grafts: synthesis, characterization and platelet adhesion study. Biomaterials **20**(10): 943 – 953 (1999)

23. Lim, F., C. Z. Yang, S. L. Cooper. Synthesis, characterization and ex vivo evaluation of polydimethylsiloxane polyurea-urethanes. Biomaterials **15**(6): 408 – 416 (1994)

11.10　Problems

1. What are the differences between HDPE and UHMWPE?
2. Why introducing certain sizes of pores are important in fabricating certain types of implants?
3. Why pores HDPE implants are malleable in hot water?
4. What are the advantages and disadvantages in using PMMA bone cement?
5. What are the possible ways to reduce the heat release of PMMA bone cement?
6. List some of the polymers which can be used to manufacture non-degradable surgical sutures.
7. How would you prepare a nylon with greater moisture resistance than Nylon-66?
8. Which would have higher melting point, (a) a polyamide or (b) polyester with similar numbers of methylene groups in the repeat units?
9. What would be an easy way to synthesise a polyurethane hydrogel?
10. What type of polyurethane is hydrolytically more stable, (a) poly(ether urethane), (b) poly(ester urethane), (c) poly(carbonate urethane)?
11. In what cases would you chose to use PEEK or polysulfone as biomaterial?
12. What are the advantages and disadvantages of using non-biodegradable polymer biomaterials?

12 Synthetic Biodegradable Polymers

Biodegradable polymers offer the advantage of being able to be eliminated from the body after fulfilling their intended use. Therefore, avoid the usual costly and complicated procedures to remove the implants or scaffolds. It is not surprising that biodegradable biomaterials are becoming more and more important in biomaterials and tissue engineering field. In this chapter, some of the important synthetic polymers will be reviewed.

12.1 Aliphatic Polyester

Aliphatic polyesters presently are the most attractive synthetic biodegradable polymers for biomedical use. These biodegradable polymers all have hydrolysable ester linkages in their structure. Table 12.1 summarizes the commonly seen biodegradable aliphatic polyesters [1].

Table 12.1　Synthetic biodegradable aliphatic polyester

Name of Polymer	Structure
Poly(glycolic acid) (PGA)	$\left[O-CH_2-CO \right]_n$
Poly(lactic acid) (PLA)	$\left[O-\overset{\displaystyle H}{\underset{\displaystyle CH_3}{C}}-CO \right]_n$
Poly(ε-caprolactone) (PCL)	$\left[O-(CH_2)_5-CO \right]_n$
Poly(para-dioxanone) (PDS)	$\left[O-(CH_2)_2-O-CH_2-CO \right]_n$
Poly(hydroxybutyrate) (PHB)	$\left[O-\underset{\displaystyle CH_3}{CH}-CH_2-CO \right]_n$
Polyvalerolactone (PVL)	$\left[O-(CH_2)_4-CO \right]_n$

12.1 Aliphatic Polyester

Continued

Name of Polymer	Structure
Poly(hydroxyvalerate) (PHV)	$\begin{array}{c} \{O-CH-CH_2-CO\}_n \\ \quad\quad\mid \\ \quad H_2C-CH_3 \end{array}$
Poly(β-malic acid) (PMLA)	$\begin{array}{c} \{O-CH-CH_2-CO\}_n \\ \quad\quad\mid \\ \quad\quad COOH \end{array}$

In theory, the synthesis of these aliphatic biodegradable polymers can also be synthesized by the step growth condensation polymerization of either hydroxyacids (See (12.1)).

$$HO-R-COOH \longrightarrow \{O-R-CO\}_n + n\,H_2O$$

(12.1)

or diols and diacids (See (12.2)).

$$HO-R-OH + HOOC-R'-COOH \longrightarrow$$

$$\{HO-R-O-CO-R'-CO\}_n + n H_2O$$

(12.2)

However, due to the difficulty in removing the small molecule by product like water, the direct polycondensation will yield low molecular weight polyesters. High molecular weight aliphatic polyesters can be synthesized by ring opening polymerization of heterocyclic monomers bearing at least one ester bond in the monomer structure (See (12.3)).

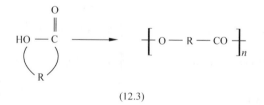

(12.3)

12.1.1 Poly(glycolide)

Poly(glycolide) (PGA) is synthesized through the ring opening polymerization of glycolide to yield high-molecular-weight materials. The monomer glycolide is synthesized from the dimerization of glycolic acid (12.4)[1,2].

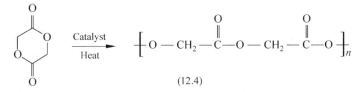

(12.4)

As shown in (12.4), PGA is the simplest linear aliphatic polyester. It is highly crystalline (45% – 55%) with a high melting point (220°C – 225°C) and a glass transition temperature of 35°C – 40°C[3]. Because of its high degree of crystallization, it is not soluble in most organic solvents except for highly fluorinated organic solvents such as hexafluoroisopropanol.

PGA Fibers exhibit high strength and modulus because of its high degree of crystallinity. But it is too stiff to be used as sutures except as braided material. PGA was used to develop the first totally synthetic absorbable suture that has been marketed as Dexon™ since the 1960s by Davis and Geck [1 – 3]. Sutures of PGA lose about 50% of their strength after two weeks and 100% after four weeks and are completely absorbed in 4 – 6 months [2].

Glycolide can be copolymerized with other monomers, such as lactide and trimethylene carbonate, to yield copolymer with various mechanical and biodegradation properties for different applications.

12.1.2 Poly(lactide)

Lactic acid is a chiral molecule, and exists in two stereo-isometric forms: D-LA and L-LA. The monomer used to synthesis poly(lactide) (PLA) is lactide, which is the cyclic dimer of lactic acid. L-lactide, is the naturally occurring isomer, and DL-lactide is the synthetic blend of D-lactide and L-lactide. The polymerization of lactide is similar to that of glycolide (12.5).

Both poly(D-LA) (PDLA) and poly(L-LA) (PLLA) are crystalline polymers.

PLLA is the most commonly used form than PDLA because the degradation product L-lactic acid is the natural occurring stereoisomer of lactic acid [4]. Poly(L-lactide) is about 37% crystalline with a melting point of 175°C –

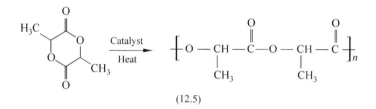

(12.5)

178 °C and a glass transition temperature of 60 °C – 65 °C [5].

Because PLLA and PDLA exhibit high tensile strengths and high modulus that makes them more applicable than the amorphous poly(DL-LA) (PDLLA) polymers for load-bearing applications such as in orthopedic fixation and sutures. However, the degradation time of PLLA is much longer than that of PDLLA. It takes more than 3 years for PLLA to be completely absorbed [6].

As a biodegradable polymer, PLLA has satisfactory biocompatibility *in vitro* [7,8]. It is essentially non-toxic, and elicits only a mild inflammatory response. The hydrolysis product L-lactic acid is the normal intermediate of carbohydrate metabolism and will not accumulate in vital organs. It has been proposed and successfully applied in the reconstruction of bone, articular defects, suture materials, drug carriers, and fixation devices [9].

However, the slow *in vivo* degradation rate of PLLA opposes a problem for its application. It has been found that bone plates made of crystalline (PLLA) were used for the fixation of zygoma fractures. After 3 years, all patients showed a severe, well-defined swelling, which was strictly limited to the implantation site. In the case of seven patients, surgeries were performed to surgically remove the swelling. Light microscopic examination showed that the removed tissue was characterized by a foreign body reaction without signs of inflammation. Examination of the tissue samples using transmission electron microscopic revealed the presence of large amounts of highly crystalline PLLA particles. Therefore, it is believed that the swelling of the implantation site was caused by the aseptic inflammatory reaction of the host tissue to the small crystalline PLLA particles. It is also confirmed that the degradation of the PLLA crystals was very slow and that the total degradation time was much longer than 3 years [10].

To overcome this problem, D-lactic acid was added as co-monomer to obtain a copolymer with a lower crystallinity than PLLA and consequently a higher degradation rate.

12. 1. 3   Poly(lactide-co-glycolide)

Lactide and glycolide can be copolymerized to obtain a range of copolymers with various mechanical and biodegradation properties (12. 6).

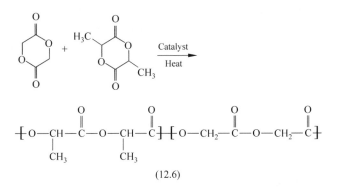

(12.6)

Copolymers of glycolide with both L-lactide and DL-lactide have been developed for both device and drug delivery applications. It has been found that there is not a linear relationship between the copolymer composition and the mechanical and degradation properties of the materials. For example, a copolymer of 50% glycolide and 50% DL-lactide degrades faster than both homopolymers [11]. The degradation rate strongly depends on the crystallinity of the copolymers. Copolymers of 25% − 70% L-lactide with glycolide are amorphous due to the disruption of the regularity of the polymer chain by the other monomer [1,2]. Therefore, these copolymer showed a much higher degradation rates than each individual homopolymers. Relationship between the copolymer composition and the mechanical and degradation properties of the materials is non-linear. For example, the degradation time of these copolymers were found to increase in the following order [1]:

$$PLA_{100}(6.7 \text{months}) < PGA(5 \text{months}) < PLA_{75}GA_{25}(2.5 \text{ weeks})$$
$$< PLA_{25}GA_{75}(2 \text{ weeks}) < PLA_{50}GA_{50}(1 \text{ week})$$

The half-life of the copolymers decreased from 5 months for PGA to 1 week for $PLA_{50}GA_{50}$ and rapidly increased to 6.7 months for PLA_{100}.

Some applications include using 82/18 poly(L-lactide-co-glycolide) copolymers as suture anchors and as screws and plates for craniomaxillofacial repair respectively [12, 13].

12.1.4 Poly(ε-caprolactone)

Poly(ε-caprolactone) (PCL) can be synthesized through the ring opening polymerization of ε-caprolactone (12.7). PCL is a semicrystalline polymer with a melting point of 59°C − 64°C and a glass-transition temperature of about 60°C. The degradation time of PCL is about two years [2]. In order to accelerate the degradation rate, DL-lactide is used to copolymerize with ε-caprolactone to yield copolymers with more rapid degradation rate. It has been found that the copolymers with 11%, 23%, 47%, and 90% mol of DL-lactide have much higher degradation rates than the corresponding homopolymers [1].

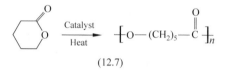

(12.7)

The structure of the copolymer will affect the degradation rate. For example, both random and block copolymers of PCL-co-DL-LA can be synthesized. It has been shown that the random copolymers degraded faster than the parent homopolymers, whereas the block copolymer degraded at an intermediate rates.

Because PCL has a low glass transition temperature, monomer ε-caprolactone has been used to copolymerize with glycolide to reduce the stiffness of pure poly(glycolide) (PGA). Such a block copolymer has been used as a monofilament suture under the trade name MONOCRYL' by Ethicon [1, 2].

12.1.5 Poly(para-dioxanone)

Poly(para-dioxanone)(PDS) is synthesized through the ring opening polymerization of p-dioxanone. This material has about 55% crystallinity with a T_m about 106°C − 115°C and glass transition temperature of −10°C to 0°C. Compared to PGA, PDS has a better flexibility because of the ether linkage in its structure. Because it contains fewer ester linkages in its molecules structure when compared to PGA and PGLA copolymers, the degradation rate of poly (para-dioxanone)(PDS) is slower both *in vitro* and *in vivo*. The degradation rate of PDS can be enhanced by incorporating of 5% −25% glycolide as comonomer [1].

Poly(dioxanone) showed no acute or toxic effects on implantation (See (12.8)).

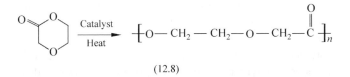

(12.8)

Poly(para-dioxanone) is mainly used as biodegradable suture materials. Other aplications include absorbable pin for fracture fixations [2].

12. 2   Poly(propylene fumarate)

Poly(propylene fumarate) (PPF) is an alternative copolymer of propylene glycol and fumaric acid. The synthesis of PPF is illustrated in (12.9). Briefly, monomer di-(2-hydroxypropyl) fumarate is first synthesized by the reaction of fumaryl chloride with propylene glycol in methylene chloride. Then PPF is synthesized by a transesterification reaction between the monomer di-(2-hydroxypropyl) fumarate molecules at high temperature [14].

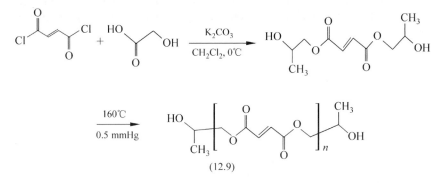

(12.9)

PPF has ester linkages in its structure. Therefore, PPF can be hydrolyzed through a hydrolysis mechanism. The unsaturated double bond in its structure unit makes it possible to be crosslinked through radical polymerization. The structure units propylene glycol fumaric acid can be excreted via normal metabolic pathways. Fumaric acid is a component of Krebs cycle, and propylene glycol has been used as an intravenous fluid component.

This polymer was developed mainly as an injectable bone cement [15]. The main advantage of this unsaturated polymer is the ability to cure the material *in vivo*, thereby filling the skeleton defect of any shape or size with minimal surgical intervention. PPF can be cured or crosslinked using a vinyl monomer, such as *N*-vinyl pyrrolidone (NVP), with a radical initiating system such as benzoyl peroxide/dimethyl toluidine. Changing the PPF to vinyl monomer ratio can change the ultimate mechanical properties and the degradation rate of cured polymer.

In vivo studies have demonstrated that NVP cross-linked PPF is a biocompatible biodegradable polymer. There is significant bone ingrowth into the polymer at 5 weeks post-implantation in a rat proximal tibia model study.

12.3 Polyamino Acid

The idea of using polyamino acid is that the peptide linkage can be broken down enzymatically. The degradation products then would be amino acids and polypeptide, which should be utilized by the body. However, when using polyamino acid as biodegradable materials, the antigenicity of the polyamino acid with more than 3 amino acids in their structure is a concern. Therefore, polyamino acids with single type of amino acid, such as poly(L-lysine), poly-L-glutamic acid, were synthesized. These polymers are difficult to process because of their high crystallinity. To overcome these problems, a modified "pseudo" poly(amino acids) has been synthesized using a tyrosine derivative.

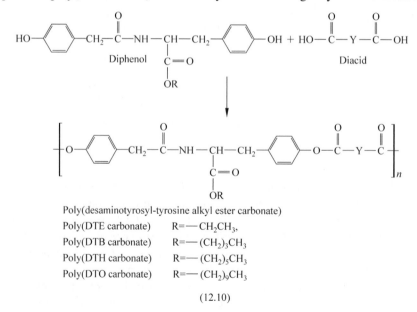

Poly(desaminotyrosyl-tyrosine alkyl ester carbonate)
Poly(DTE carbonate)   R=—CH$_2$CH$_3$,
Poly(DTB carbonate)   R=—(CH$_2$)$_3$CH$_3$
Poly(DTH carbonate)   R=—(CH$_2$)$_5$CH$_3$
Poly(DTO carbonate)   R=—(CH$_2$)$_9$CH$_3$

(12.10)

Tyrosine-derived polycarbonates are high strength materials that may be useful as orthopedic implants [4].

The tyrosine-based polycarbonate poly(DTE carbonate) showed significant bone apposition when implanted in a bony site [16].

12.4 References

1. Li, S., M. Vert. Biodegradation of aliphatic polyesters. In: Gerald Scott and Dan Gilead, eds. Degradation Polymers. Chapman & Hall, London, pp. 43 –87 (1995)
2. Middleton, J. C., A. J. Tipton. Synthetic biodegradable polymers as orthopedic devices. Biomaterials **21**: 2335 –2346 (2000)
3. Shalaby, S. W., R. A. Johnson. Synthetic absorbable polyesters. In: S. W. Shalaby, ed. Biomedical polymers. Designed to degrade systems. New York, Hanser, pp. 1 –34 (1994)
4. Kohn, J., R. Langer. Bioresorbable and bioerodible materials. In: B. D. Ratner, A. S. Hoffman, F. J. Schoen, J. E. Lemons, (eds), Biomaterials Science. New York, Academic Press, pp. 64 –72 (1996)
5. Daniels, A. U., M. K. O Chang, K. P Andriano, J. Heller. Mechanical properties of biodegradable polymers and composites proposed for internal fixation of bone. J. Appl. Biomater. **1**: 57 –78 (1990)
6. Bergsma, J. E., W. C. de Bruijn, F. R. Rozema, R. R. M. Bos, G. Boering. Late degradation tissue response to poly(L-lactide) bone plates and screws. Biomaterials. **16**(1): 25 –31 (1995)
7. Sliedregt, A. van, K. de Groot, C. A. van Blitterswijk. In Vitro biocompatibility testing of polylactides. Part I: Proliferation of different cell types. J. Mater. Sci: Mater. in Med. **3**: 365 –370 (1992)
8. van Sliedregt, A., K. de Groot, C. A. van Blitterswijk. In Vitro biocompatibility testing of polylactides. Part II. J. Mater. Sci: Mater. in Med. **4**: 213 (1993)
9. Verheyen, C. C. P. M., J. R. de Wijn, C. A. van Blitterswijk, K. de Groot. Evaluation of hydroxyapatite/poly(L-lactide) composites: mechanical behavior, J. Biomed. Mater. Res. **26**: 1277 –1296 (1992)
10. Bergsma, E. J., F. R. Rozema, R. R. Bos, W. C. de Bruijn. Foreign body reactions to resorbable poly(L-lactide) bone plates and screws used for the fixation of unstable zygomatic fractures. J. Oral. Maxillofac. Surg. **51**(6): 666 –670 (1993)
11. Miller, R. A., J. M. Brady, D. E. Cutright. Degradation rates of oral resorbable implants (polylactates and polyglycolates): rate modification with changes in PLA/PGA copolymer ratios. J. Biomed. Mater. Res. **11**: 711 –719 (1977)
12. Gilding, D. K., A. M. Reed. Biodegradable polymers for use in surgery-polyglycolic/poly(lactic acid) homo- and copolymers: 1. Polymer **20**: 1459 (1964)
13. Pietrzak, W. S., B. S. Verstynen, D. R. Sarver. Bioabsorbable fixation devices: status for the craniomaxillofaxial surgeon. J. Craniofaxial Surg. **2**: 92 – 96 (1997)
14. He, S., M. D. Timmer, M. J. Yaszemski, A. W. Yasko, P. S. Engel, A. G. Mikos. Synthesis of biodegradable poly(propylene fumarate) networks with poly(propylene fumarate) diacrylate macromers as crosslinking agents and characterization of their degradation products. Polymer **42**: 1251 – 1260 (2001)

15. Peter, S. J., P. Kim, A. W. Yasko, M. J. Yaszemski, A. G. Mikos. Crosslinking characteristics of an injectable poly(propylene fumarate)/β-tricalcium phosphate paste and mechanical properties of the crosslinked composite for use as a biodegradable bone cement. J. Biomed. Mater. Res. **44**: 314 – 321 (1999)
16. James, K., H. Levene, E. E. Kaufmann, J. R. Parsons, J. Kohn. Small changes in chemical structure of a polymer can have a significant effect on the hard-tissue response *in vivo*. In: J. E. Davies, ed. Bone Engineering. EM Squared Inc. Toronto, Canada, pp. 195 – 203 (2000)

12.5 Problems

1. Give the basic chemical structure for the following polymers: polyethylene, polypropylene, polystyrene, polyurethane, PDMS, and PGLA.
2. List 5 applications for biodegradable polymers.
3. What are the advantages of using biodegradable polymers?
4. In what cases would you choose to use biodegradable polymer rather than use non-biodegradable polymers?
5. If you need to use a polymer should be a totally degraded *in vivo* within a few weeks, what kind of polymer would you chose?
6. Why PDS is more flexible than PGA?
7. If you need to design a flexible totally biodegradable implant, what polymer would you use?
8. Can you design a totally biodegradable bone cement?
9. What are the advantages and disadvantages of using poly(amino acid) as biomaterials?
10. What is the most effective way to change the degradation rate of a polymer?
11. How will the crystallinity of a polymer affect its degradation rate?
12. What is the difference between the degradation mechanism of PLGA and poly(DTE carbonate)?

13　Polymer Matrix Composite Biomaterials

A composite material is a material consisting of two or more chemically distinct constituents, on a macroscale, having a distinct interface separating them. In practice, polymer matrix composites consist of fiber and particulate reinforced composites as biomaterials.

Most of the composite materials are designed to provide improved mechanical properties such as strength, stiffness, toughness and fatigue resistance. Therefore, they are frequently used as biomaterials for orthopaedic applications where mechanical properties are a serious concern.

Much effort has been invested in the development of composite biomaterials for the repair or replacement of hard tissue. Besides the general consideration of biocompatibility, the specific consideration for bone replacement materials is of biomechanical nature: the biomaterials should possess the mechanical properties necessary for a proper performance in their function. Other properties, such as biodegradation and the ability to bond to bone (so-called "bone-bonding" property), are some additional favourable assets. The bone bonding property can be defined as "the establishment by physicochemical processes of a continuity between implant and bone matrix" [1]. Bone bonding properties— often called "bioactivity" — have been proven to be of great benefit for bone replacement materials.

The use of polymer matrix composites for bone replacement may offer the advantages of avoiding the problem of stress shielding (a problem encountered when using high modulus metal implants), eliminating the need for a second surgical procedure to remove the implants if the implants can be biodegradable and eliminating the ion release problem of metal implants. The possibility to make the composites as strong as cortical bone and to improve the material's bioactivity or bone bonding activity by adding a secondary reinforcing phase makes the composites very attractive. Fibers and ceramic filler particles have been used to reinforce the polymer materials as well as to improve the bone-bonding properties of the composites.

13. 1   Fiber Reinforced Composites

Carbon fiber, aramid (Kevelar), and glass fiber usually possess very high strength and stiffness and therefore have been frequently used to reinforce polymers such as epoxy resin, polyetheretherketone (PEEK), polysulfone (PS), polymethyl methacrylate (PMMA), poly(lactide), poly(glycolide), polycaprolactone, etc. (Table 13. 1) [2].

Table 13. 1   Examples of fiber reinforced composites for bone replacement [2]

Fiber	Polymer Matrix
Carbon fiber	Epoxy resin, PMMA, polysulfone, polycarbonate, polyetheretherketone, polylactide.
Aramid (Kevelar)	PMMA, polysulfone, polycarbonate
Polyethylene fiber (high-performance)	PMMA, poly(DL-lactic acid)
Bioactive glass fiber	Polysulfone
Calcium metaphosphate glass fiber	Polylactide
Calcium phosphate glass fiber	Poly(L-lactide), polycaprolactone, Poly-(de-samino-tyrosyl-tyrosine ethyl ester)
Titanium fiber	PMMA
Calcium-sodium-metaphosphate glass fiber	Poly(ortho ester)

By proper choice of the type of polymer matrix and the fiber, the composites can be made totally biodegradable, partially degradable, or non-biodegradable. Also the mechanical properties can be tailored by combining different polymer matrices and fibers. As an example, 30% carbon fiber reinforced PEEK composites have an elastic modulus of 17 GPa (bone 7 − 20 GPa), a flexural strength of 320 MPa (bone 150 − 250 MPa) [3].

Bone bonding can be improved by using certain bioactive fibers. It has been shown that when bioactive glass reinforced polysulfone composites were implanted for 6 weeks, direct apposition of bone tissue with bioactive glass fibers could be observed. Bone tissue was also observed in direct apposition to polymers surrounding the glass fibers [4, 5].

When making fiber reinforced composites, the mechanical properties of the polymer matrix and the fiber are certainly important for the mechanical properties of the composites. However, the interfacial bonding strength between fibers and polymer matrix is usually weaker than the polymer matrix. Therefore, the fatigue fractures usually occur at the interface of fiber and polymer.

When the composite is exposed to an *in vivo* environment, the interface of fiber and polymer can be further deteriorated. Several studies have shown the effect of water in simulated *in vivo* environments on the interfacial bonding strength of ceramic or glass fiber and polymer. These results clearly indicated that there is a need for the improvement of the interface of fiber/polymer matrix to improve both the mechanical properties of the composites and the wet stability of the interfacial bond.

13. 2   Filler Reinforced Composites

The use of particulate fillers to reinforce polymeric biomaterials is quite important and successful in clinical applications, like dental restorative resins and bone cement [6].

The purpose of using filler particles in the polymer matrix is to improve the mechanical properties such as the elastic modulus, fatigue behaviour and to improve the bioactivity or bone-bonding properties [7 – 10]. Some other benefits may also obtained by using fillers, such as to diminish the creep of the composites and to decrease the temperature rise during the polymerization of bone cements [11].

The use of bioactive filler such as hydroxyapatite (HA), AW^{TM} ceramic or Bioglass^{TM} particles to reinforce a polymer may improve both the mechanical properties and the bone bonding properties. It has been indicated [7] that the elastic modulus of polyethylene(PE) can be increased from 1 GPa to about 8 GPa, which is in the low band of the value for bone, retaining fracture toughness comparable to bone. When implanted *in vivo*, the HA/PE composites can induce bone apposition and thus create a secure bond between the natural bone and the implant. Inspired by this work, researches have been extended to the biodegradable polymer matrix. When implanted *in vivo*, such composites will induce bone formation or bone ingrowth and as the biodegradable polymer matrix degrades the implant will finally be replaced by bone tissue. The load thus can be gradually transferred to the newly formed bone. Based on this idea, several hydroxyapatite reinforced biodegradable polymer composites have been developed, such as HA/polyhydroxybutyrate [8,9], and HA/polylactide [10].

The use of a filler to reinforce a biodegradable polymer matrix offers another advantage: the possibility to control the biodegradation rate. It has been shown that by adding of basic fillers, such as HA and magnesium oxide, the degradation rate as well as the degradation mechanism of poly (DL-lactide) and poly(L-lactide) can be changed [12, 13].

13.3 Methods to Improve the Interfacial Bonding Between Phases in Composites

13.3.1 Self-Reinforcement of Fiber/Polymer Composites

Compared to its bulk polymer material, polymer fibers usually possess much better mechanical properties due to their molecular orientation. Use of polymer fibers to reinforce a polymer matrix of the same chemical structure thus will result in a composite without a real interface between fibers and polymer matrix. Such self-reinforced composites have been made by using Poly (lactic acid) (PLA) [14], Poly(glycolic acid) (PGA) [15, 16] and polymethyl methacrylate(PMMA) [17]. The mechanical properties of the composites were significantly improved by using this method. However, the polymer fibers used are still pliable, therefore, the Young's moduli of SRC's cannot be as high as those of glass fiber and carbon fiber reinforced composites. On the other hand, the bone bonding properties of the composites cannot be improved by this method.

13.3.2 Plasma Treatment of Fibers

Gas plasma treatment has been proven to be effective in enhancing the bond strength between fibers and polymer matrix. The gas used for the treatment of fiber can be argon gas, O_2, methane or CO_2. These methods have been used to treat fibers like polyethylene, calcium phosphate glass fiber and polylethylene terephthalate(PET) (Table 13.2).

Table 13.2 Examples of using gas plasma treatment for the improvement of fiber/matrix interface [2]

Fiber	Gas	Matrix
Polyethylene	Air	Poly(DL-lactic acid)
	N_2, Ar, CO_2	PMMA
PET	Ar, O_2	PMMA
Calcium-phosphate glass fiber	CH_4	Poly (desaminotyrosyl-tyrosine alkyl ester carbonate)

During the gas plasma treatment, functional groups are generated on the surface of the fiber. Therefore the wettability of the fibers by the polymer matrix and thus the bond strength between them is improved.

13.3.3   Coupling Agent

A coupling agent is an additive, which promotes the development of a strong bond between the filler (fiber) surface and the polymer. Over the years, researchers have developed several coupling agents, which can improve the interfacial bonding in the composites.

13.3.3.1   Silane Coupling Agents

Silane coupling agents have been widely used to improve the bonding strength of the two phases and have a general formula as:

$$X_3SiRY$$

X represents a hydrolysable group, Y is a organo functional group. The organo functional groups are chosen for reactivity or compatibility with the polymer, while the hydrolysable groups are merely intermediate in the formation of a bond with the filler or fiber surface. The exact behaviour of coupling agent is a matter of some controversy.

The use of silane coupling agents in mineral filled dental resins has been employed since the 1960's as a method to improve the bonding of the filler to the resin. It was reported that appropriate silane coupling agents were chosen for a variety of mineral fillers to improve the mechanical properties of composites [18]. The greatest improvement was observed with silica, alumina, glass, silicon carbide, and aluminum needles. A good but somewhat lesser response was observed with talc, wollastonite, iron powder, clay, and hydrated aluminum oxide. Only a slight improvement was imparted to asbestine, hydroxyapatite(HA), titanium dioxide, and zinc oxide. Surfaces that showed little or no apparent response to silane coupling agents included calcium carbonate, graphite and boron. Those results suggest that the coupling activity of silanes is not universal to all mineral surfaces.

The effect of the use of silane coupling agents on HA seems to have somewhat controversial results. It has been shown that silane treated with HA particles have a positive effect on the mechanical properties of a composite. Some researchers [19] have shown that applying methacryloxypropyltrimethoxysilane (MPS) to the surface of HA particles may enhance the tensile modulus, yield stress and elongation to fracture of polyethylmethacrylate cements. Using MPS also significantly improved the hardness, flexural strength and diametral tensile strength of dental composites [20].

However, silane coupling agents also have been found to have different effect on the mechanical properties of other composites. Some researchers [21, 22] found that MPS treated HA showed decreased tensile strength and Young's modulus of polyethylene composite. Since in both cases there was no chemical bonding between the silane and the polymer matrix, the decreased strength and modulus was explained by a plasticizing effect of the coupling agent. Surface treatment of β-crystalline metaphosphate with silane coupling agent MPS did not have effect on the tensile strength of dental resin composites [23].

13.3.3.2 Ionic Polymer Coupling Agents

In an effort to improve the adhesion of HA filler particles to a polyethylene/poly(butylenes terephathalate) block copolymer matrix (Polyactive^{TM}), ionic bonding and hydrogen bonding were introduced to the interfaces between HA filler particles and Polyactive^{TM} matrix by using polyacrylic acid (PAA) and ethylene-maleic acid (EMA) copolymer. It is well known that PAA and EMA can be firmly adsorbed onto the surface of HA. On the other hand, PAA and EMA can also form hydrogen bond with polyethylene glycol which is presented in the structure of Polyactive^{TM}. Therefore, the adhesion of HA particles to the polymer matrix was enhanced by the presence of PAA or EMA at the interface. The mechanical properties of the resulting composites were significantly improved both in dry and wet state. Scanning electron microscopy(SEM) studies showed that HA filler particles modified with PAA or EMA adhered better to the polymer matrix [24, 25].

13.3.3.3 Isocyanate Coupling Agents

Isocyanate reagents were studied as coupling agents in nano sized HA (nanoapatite) reinforced polymer composites. It was found that isocyanates were able to chemically bond to the surface of HA [26, 27]. Therefore, isocyanate and diisocyanates can be used to introduce chemical bonding between HA particles and the various polymer matrix. By using this method, polyethylene glycol, poly (methyl methacrylate) (PMMA), poly (hydroxyehtyl methacrylate) (PHEMA), and poly(butyl methacrylate) (PBMA) were covalently bond to the HA particles [28]. Similarly, using hexamehtylene diisocyanate as coupling agent, covalent bonding between HA filler particles and polymer matrix could be achieved and the mechanical properties of the composites were greatly improved in wet state [29].

13.3.3.4   Other Methods

It was found that 4-methacryloyloxyethyl trimellitic anhydride (4-META) containing methyl methacrylate(MMA) bone cement could adhere to bone, metals, HA and a composite of HA and fluoroapatite (FAP) with a improved tensile bond strength [30]. The bonding of such cement to dentin was explained by the ability of 4-META to promote the interpenetration of monomers into dentin tissue. No explanation was given to the adhesiveness of such cements to HA and metals. Some researchers speculate that the formation of 4-methacryloyloxyethyl trimellitic acid (4-MET) was the reason of adhesion to HA. The anhydride moiety of 4-META can be easily converted to 4-MET by the reaction with water, thus the real mechanism might either be that 4-MET is firmly absorbed to the surface of HA followed by the copolymerization of 4-MET with MMA monomer, or the copolymerization takes place first and is followed by the adsorption of 4-MET moieties onto HA. In both cases, the interface of HA and polymer may be improved. Therefore, using 4-MET is similar to the use of ionic polymers as coupling agents [2].

Zirconates have been studied as coupling agents. It has been found that [31] when the HA surface had been surface treated with zirconyl methacrylate, the diametral tensile strength of dental composites was increased by 50%. It was also found that [23] treatment of fillers by zirconyl methacrylate resulted in a modest enhancement of the tensile strength of the experimental composites.

Introduction of covalently bonded hydroxyethylmethacrylate (HEMA) to a nonstoichiometric apatitic calcium phosphate was realized by a co-precipitation of apatitic octacalcium phosphate (AOCP) in the presence of hydroxyethylmethacrylate phosphate [32]. The bond of the organic HEMA to AOCP was realized by the ionized phosphate groups, which partially replace the OH-ions located at the tunnel end in the apatite crystal structure. The obtained so-called phospho HEMA apatite can then be used to co-polymerize with either HEMA or methyl methacrylate (MMA) to form chemical bonds between the mineral filler and the polymer matrix. It is claimed that such filler could stiffen the PMMA bone cement.

13.4   References

1.   William, D. F., J. Black, P. J. Doherty. Second consensus conference on definitions in biomaterials. In: P. J. Doherty, R. L. Williams, D. F. Williams, A. J. C. Lee, eds., Advances in Biomaterials: Biomaterial-tissue Interfaces. 10, Elsevier Science

13.4 References

Publishers, Amsterdam, pp. 525 – 533 (1992)

2. Liu, Q., Hydroxyapatite/polymer Composites for Bone Replacement. Chapter 1, Ph. D. Thesis, Twente University (1987)
3. Hastings, R. S., S. A. Brown, A. Moet. Characterization of short fiber reinforced polymers for fracture fixation device. Trans. Soc. Biomater: **10**: 262 (1987)
4. Marcolongo, M., P. Ducheyne, J. Garino. Interfacial bond strength between bioactive glass fiber/polymer composite and bone tissue. Trans. Soc. Biomater. **18**: 374 (1995)
5. Marcolongo, M., P. Ducheyne, E. Schepers, J. Garino. The "Halo" effect : surface reactions of a bioactive galss fiber/polymeric composite *in vitro* and *in vivo*. Trans. 5th World Biomaterials Congress, Toronto, pp. Ⅱ – 444 (1996)
6. Soltesz, U., Ceramics in composites, review and current status. In: P. Ducheyne, J. E. Lemons eds. Bioceramics: materials characteristics versus in vivo behavior. Annals of New York Academy of Sciences. **523**: pp. 137 – 156 (1988)
7. Bonfield, W., C. Doyle, K. E. Tanner. *In vivo* evaluation of hydroxyapatite reinforced polyethylene composites. In: P. Christel, A. Meunier, A. J. C. Lee eds., Biological and Biomedical Performance of Biomaterials. Elsevier, Amsterdam, pp. 153 – 159 (1986)
8. Doyle, C., K. E. Tanner, W. Bonfield. *In vitro* and *in vivo* evaluation of polyhydroxybutyrate and of polyhydroxybutyrate reinforced with hydroxyapatite. Biomaetrials **12**: 841 – 847 (1991)
9. Knowles, J. C., G. W. Hastings, H. Ohta, S Niwa, N. Boeree. Development of a degradable composite for orthopaedic use: in vivo biomedical and histological evaluation of two bioactive degradable composites based on the polyhydroxybutyrate polymer. Biomaterials **13**: 491 – 496 (1992)
10. Verheyen, C. C. P. M., J. R. de Wijn, C. A. van Blitterswijk, K. de Groot, P. M. Rozing. Hydroxyapatite/poly (L-lactide composites: an animal study on push-out strengths and interface histology. J. Biomed. Mater. Res. **27**: 433 – 444 (1993)
11. Guida, G., V. Riccio, S. Gatto, C. Migliaresi, L. Nicodemo, L. Nicolais, C. Palomba. A glass bead composite acrylic bone cement. In: P. Ducheyne, G. van der Perre, A. E. Aubert eds. Biomaterials and Biomechanics 1983, Elsevier Science Publishers B. V., Amsterdam, pp. 19 – 24 (1984)
12. van, der Meer S. A. T., J. R. de Wijn, J. G. C. Wolke. The influence of basic filler materials on the degradation of amorphous D- and L-lactide copolymer. J. Mater. Sci. : Mater. in Med. **7**: 359 – 361 (1996)
13. Jones, N. L., D. F. Williams. Poly (L-lactide) and poly (L-lactide)-ceramic fillered composites: a long term *in vivo/in vitro* degradation study. Trans. 5th World Biomaterials Congress. Toronto, pp. Ⅱ – 441 (1996)
14. Vainionpaa, S., A. Majola, M. Mero, K. Vihtonen, A. Makela, J. Vasenus, P. Rokkanen, P. Tormala. Biodegradation and biocompatibility of the polylactic acid in bone tissue and mechanical properties in vitro. Trans. Soc. Biomater. **11**: 500 (1988)
15. Laiho, J., T. Mikkonen, P. Tormala. A comparison of in vitro degradation of biodegradable polyglycolide (PGA) sutures and rods. Trans. Soc. Biomater. **11**: 564 (1988)
16. Pellinen, M., T. Pohjonen, M. Tamminmaki, P, Helevirta, P. Tormala. The *in vitro* degradation of biodegradable self-reinforced (SR) polyglycolide rods. Trans. Soc. Biomater. **11**: 562 (1988)

17. Gilbert, J. J., D. S. Ney, E. P. Lautenschlager. Self-reinforced composite poly(methyl methacrylate): static and fatigue properties. Biomaterails **16**: 1043 – 1055 (1995)

18. Plueddemann, E. P., *Silane Coupling Agents,* 2nd Edition, Plenum Press, New York, p. 118 (1991)

19. Behiri, J. C., M. Braden, S. N. Khorasani, D. Wiwattanadate, W. Bonfield. Advanced bone cement for long term orthopaedic implantations. Bioceramics **4**: 301 – 307 (1991)

20. Labella, R., M. Braden, S. Deb. Novel hydroxyapatite based dental composites. Biomaterals **15**: 1197 – 1200 (1994)

21. Deb, S., M. Wang, K. E. Tanner, W. Bonfield. Hydroxyapatite-polyethylene composites: effect of grafting and surface treatment of hydroxyapatite. J. Mater. Sci.: Mater. in Med. **7**: 191 – 193 (1996)

22. Nazhat, S. N., R. Smith, S. Deb, M. Wang, K. E. Tanner, W. Bonfield. Dynamic mechanical behaviour of modified hydroxyapatite reinforced polyethylene composites. Trans. 5th World Biomaterials Congress. Toronto, pp. II – 83 (1996)

23. Antonucci, J. M., B. O. Fowler, S. Venz. Filler systems based on calcium metaphosphates. Dent. Mater. **7**: 124 – 129 (1991)

24. Liu, Q., J. R. de Wijn, D. Bakker, C. A. van Blitterswijk. Surface modification of hydroxyapatite to introduce interfacial bonding with Polyactive™ 70/30 in a biodegradable composite. J. Mater. Sci.: Mater. in Med. **7**: 551 – 557(1996)

25. Liu, Q., J. R. de Wijn, D. Bakker, M. v. Toledo, C. A. van Blitterswijk. Polyacids as bonding agents in hydroxyapatite/polyester-ether (Polyactive™ 30/70) composites. J. Mater. Sci.: Mater. in Med. **9**: 23 – 30 (1998)

26. Liu, Q., J. R. de Wijn, C. A. van Blitterswijk. A study on the grafting reaction of isocyanates with hydroxyapatite particles. J. Biomd. Mater. Res. **40**: 358 – 364 (1998)

27. Liu, Q., J. R. de Wijn, K. de Groot, C. A. van Blitterswijk. Surface modification of nano-apatite by grafting organic polymers. Biomaterials **19**: 1067 – 1072 (1998)

28. Liu, Q., J. R. de Wijn, C. A. van Blitterswijk. Covalent bonding of PMMA, PBMA and poly(HEMA) to hydroxyapatite particles. J. Biomedical Materials Research **40**: 257 – 263 (1998)

29. Liu, Q., J. R. de Wijn, C. A. van Blitterswijk. Composite biomaterials with chemical bonding between hydroxyapatite filler particles and PEG/PBT block copolymer matrix. J. Biomed. Mater. Res. **40**: 490 – 491 (1998)

30. Ishhara, K., H. Arai, N. Nakabayashi. Adhesive bone cement containing hydoxyapatite particle as bone compatible filler. J. Biomed. Mater. Res. **26**: 937 – 945 (1992)

31. Misra, D. N., Adsorption of zirconyl salts and their acids on hydroxyapatite: use of salts as coupling agents to dental polymer composites. J. Dental. Res. **12**: 1405 – 1408 (1985)

32. Dandurand, J., V. Delpech, A. Lebugle, A. Lamure, C. Lacabanne. Study of the mineral-organic linkage in an apatitic reinforced bone cement. J. Biomed. Mater. Res. **24**: 1377 – 1384 (1990)

13.5 Problems

1. What is the main "ceramic" material found in bone?
2. What is a composite?
3. What are the main advantages and disadvantages of using composites?
4. Give 4 examples of natural composites?
5. How to turn a non-bioactive polymer material into a bioactive material?
6. Why there is a need to do the surface treatment on filler particles before making composites?
7. What is a coupling agent?
8. What kinds of interactions a coupling agent can introduce to the interface of filler/polymer matrix?
9. What is the potential impact of coupling agent on the bone bonding property of composites?
10. Please design a totally degradable composites system for none load bearing bone replacement application using a ceramic filler and a polymer?
11. How would you make a bone-replacement material X-ray-opaque?
12. Why is a good interfacial bonding between the filler surface and the resin matrix essential?

Part III

Tissue Engineering: A New Era of Regenerative Medicine[*]

* Authors of Part III are Xuejun Wen and Ning Zhang.

The lack of tissue and organs available for transplantation, as well as the problems associated with their transplantation such as donor site morbidity, immune rejection, and pathogen transfer, led to the emergence of the discipline of tissue engineering. The ultimate goal of tissue engineering as a treatment concept is to replace and even recover the anatomic structures and functions of the damaged, injured, or missing tissue and organs [1, 2].

Tissue engineering as a science discipline is the second generation of biomimetic science. It is mainly based on mimicking the *in vivo* environment *in vitro* in order to grow real tissue or tissue-like complex structures *in vitro* or *ex vivo*[1, 2]. Tissue engineering is an advanced stage of biomaterials science as well. The big improvement of tissue engineering from traditional biomaterials science is that tissue engineering is the combination of both artificial components (i.e. biomaterials) and biological components (i.e. cells, tissues, and biomolecules) to create analogues of normal tissue and organs. In contrast, traditional biomaterial science uses only artificial constructs to replace part of the normal functions of tissue and organs, rather than their anatomical structures. Therefore, tissue engineering requires various components including regeneration-component cells, carriers or support scaffolds, growth factors, and dynamic forces. Cell components are utilized to replace the previous cell loss; continuous perfusion culture is used to mimic cardiac circulation; and three-dimensional scaffolds are employed to recreate the appropriate spatial arrangement of cells in tissue and organs [3]. In summary, the fundamental approaches of tissue engineering are obtaining pieces of living tissue, disassembling the tissue into a cell suspension and expanding them to a certain concentration, seeding the cells into biocompatible scaffolds, supplying growth factors and dynamic forces to the cells, and engineering artificial tissue and organs with the anatomically desired architecture and normal functions to recover the lost body functions.

Tissue engineering as a discipline is very young and still in the early developmental stage. As such, there are lots of unknown mechanisms left to be investigated in this field. For instance, before attempting to grow any fully functional normal tissue *in vitro* or *ex vivo*, the precise mechanisms of normal tissue formation must be well understood. However, the appropriate physical, mechanical, chemical, and biological cues in normal tissue formation are currently far from understood. So do the knowledge on the environmental cues in engineering the functional tissue. Surprisingly, after only approximately four decades of growth, the field of tissue engineering is no longer limited to the academic laboratory but is rapidly growing in industry as well. For example, tissue-engineered skin is already available on market shelves in many countries including the United States and the United Kingdom [4]; tissue-engineered cartilage, temporary liver-assistance devices, and tissue-engineered pancreas are all in clinical trials [5, 6]. Up to now, investigators have attempted to grow bone [5], liver [6, 7], arteries [8], bladder [9], pancreas [10], nerves [11], cartilage [5], heart valves [8], corneas [12], and various other soft tissues [13].

Despite significant progress in both academic research and in the industry, a number of issues have arisen that have forced the research progress and commercial procedures to slow down. The biggest setback that the field of tissue engineering faces now is the unknown fate of tissue-engineered analogues inside the human body. That is why the FDA has approved only one tissue-engineered product, skin, so far. Before any further breakthroughs can be made, the following questions must be answered. Where will the transplanted cells go? How will they grow? What will they differentiate into? How will they be eliminated if an unexpected event occurs, such as tumor genesis? Unfortunately, most scientists are concentrating on regenerating all kinds of tissue and organs, but are ignoring the control issues for proper regeneration and the fate of tissue engineered grafts *in vivo*. Another problem in tissue engineering research is that most people simply seed all kinds of cells on highly porous scaffolds and expect to grow tissues with the desired structure and functions. However, they typically ignore the interactions that exist between different cell types, such as the communication between cells and the surrounding scaffold, the relationship between cells and various soluble factors, and the complex behavior of cells under physical forces, such as shear stresses, tensile and compressive loads, and vibrational forces. All these factors affect to some extent the final tissue structure. To gain further knowledge in this area, all levels of the constructed tissue structure must be well controlled and investigated. For example, organ scale scaffolds with subcellular resolution at the $1-10$ μm scale, cell level structures at the $10-100$ μm scale, and supercellular structures over 100 μm size, are to be developed. This may allow for the cellular environment, cell-scaffold communication, cell-cell interactions, and the functional unit of the tissue to be well controlled. After fully understanding these basic mechanisms, the combining of functioning cells to three-dimensional scaffolds, the regeneration of functional tissues *in vitro* and *ex vivo*, and the integration of the regenerated tissue into patients with the appropriate amount of vascularization and a controlled immune response would be easy to achieve.

14　Biomaterials for Tissue Engineering

14. 1　General Aspects of Biomaterials Used for Tissue Engineering

Biomaterials are artificial materials utilized to repair, assist, or replace damaged or missing tissue or organs. Like any other industrial material, biomaterials can be classified into four different categories: metals, ceramics, polymers, and composites. In order for any material to be considered a biomaterial, it must satisfy certain physical, mechanical, and chemical behavior requirements and also be biocompatible. For example, the material must be strong enough to bear physiological loads, be resistant to undesired degradation or corrosion, not be carcinogenic, immunogenic, antileukotactic, or mutagenic, and so on. Many factors, such as implant size, shape, material composition, surface wettability, roughness, and charge influence implant biocompatibility [2, 5, 14].

Currently, metals have been extensively used in orthopedic applications, as discussed in metallic biomaterials chapter, especially for bone and dental replacements. However, there are very few uses of metals as tissue engineering scaffolds, due to their non-degradability and undesirable mechanical properties when compared with normal tissue.

Ceramics are inorganic materials primarily used in tissue engineering to serve as supporting scaffolds for cell culture and hard tissue formation and as carriers for bioactive molecule delivery [15 – 17]. Of the many ceramics produced, the two most prominent ones that are utilized for tissue engineering, owing to their bioactivity and bio-resorbability in the body, are hydroxyapatite and bioactive glasses such as Bioglass®, which contains SiO_2, Na_2O, CaO, and P_2O_5 in specific proportions [18].

Polymers are organic and the major compositional elements, which are similar to that of the human body, are carbon, hydrogen, oxygen, nitrogen, sulfur, and phosphorus. Due to differences in elemental arrangements and production methods, polymers are the most diverse type of materials with varying mechanical and physical properties and different levels of chemical reactivity and degradation. Owing to these differences, polymers are the most popular materials used for tissue engineering [19, 20]. Specifically, biodegradable polymers show the most promising results for use as scaffolds and three categories of biodegradable polymers are the most frequently studied [3, 7, 19 –21]:

(1) FDA-approved biodegradable and bioresorbable polymers, including natural and synthetic polymers, such as collagen, polyglycolide (PGA), poly-lactide (PLA), polycaprolactone (PCL), etc. ;

(2) non-approved polymers, such as polyorthoester (POE), polyan-hydrides, etc. ; and

(3) customized degradable polymers, which can selectively bind specific cell types and ward off unwanted cell types.

Composite materials are composed of at least two different categories of materials. The composites used for tissue engineering usually consist of polymers and ceramics. The typical composites are a mixture of hydroxyapatite or Bioglass® with biodegradable polymers, such as polyesters [22]. The major application of these scaffolds is use for hard tissue engineering [22].

14. 2   Representative Biomaterials Used for Tissue Engineering

14. 2. 1   Polymers

From the origin point of view, there are two categories: natural and synthetic polymers. From the lifetime point of view, there are two categories as well: biodegradable and non-biodegradable polymers. The mostly used natural polymers are collagens and the most widely employed synthetic polymers are poly (α-hydroxy acids).

(1) Collagen — Collagen is a natural extracellular matrix (ECM) molecule found in many tissues such as bone, skin, tendons, ligaments, and other connective tissues. It has a fibrillar structure with a fiber diameter ranging from 50 nm to 500 nm [23]. Collagen provides a substrate for cellular recognition and promotes cell attachment, proliferation, and differentiated function. Cellular recognition is an advantage for promoting cell adhesion, migration, and proliferation. However, sometimes advantages can be disadvantages. For example, cellular recognition can cause immunogenicity, which is not desirable and a common problem with natural polymers. Other problems with natural polymers are inconsistencies in their mechanical properties, their degradability, and their reproducibility between samples [23, 24].

(2) Poly(α-hydroxy acid) — Poly(α-hydroxy acids) are a group of synthetic polymers. Some of them are approved by the FDA for their use in surgical sutures and a few implantable devices. Some aliphatic polyesters, such as PLA, PGA, and their co-polymers, are not only biocompatible but also biodegradable [25, 26]. In general, for regularly sized devices, aliphatic polyesters undergo a bulk degradation process. If the sample size is very large, e.g. the smallest dimension is larger than five centimeters, then the aliphatic polyester may undergo a surface erosion process. Although the major degradation mechanism of aliphatic polyesters is hydrolysis, the degradation rate of different aliphatic polyesters is different. For example, it takes about two years for 80 kDa (1 Da = 1 n) molecular weight (MW) polycaprolactone to completely dissolve, but only approximately 3 weeks for 40 kDa MW PLGA to disappear [25 – 27]. Because the major degradation products of aliphatic polyesters are acids, the massive release of acid may surpass the capacity of the surrounding tissue to eliminate it, and this may cause an elevated inflammatory reaction. In particular, if there is poor vascularization at the implantation site, the local environment may be seriously disturbed. Chang and other researchers have studied mixing basic bioceramics, such as tricalcium phosphate (TCP) and hydroxyapatite (HA), into polyesters to buffer the acidic by-products. The bioceramic-polyester composite can not only avoid the formation of an unfavorable pH environment for the cells, but can also improve the capacity of the environment to promote bone tissue regeneration [25, 26]. The other problem with pure synthetic polymers is the lack of cellular recognition and therefore difficult to make dynamic communication between synthetic materials and cells. One way to overcome this problem is grafting the short functional peptides on the surface of synthetic polymers [28 – 30].

14.2.2   Bioceramics

Bioceramics, particularly calcium phosphates and bioactive glasses, have shown very promising results in hard tissue regeneration applications owing to their high bioactivity and their formation of interfacial chemical bonds with host tissue, i.e. osseointegration.

Calcium phosphate ceramics are chemically similar to the mineral component of bones and other hard tissues in mammals, i.e. they are composed of the same ions that make up the mineral constituents of teeth and bones. They show excellent biocompatibility with not only hard tissues, but also with skin and muscle tissues, without any toxic effects [16, 18]. Unfortunately, their mechanical properties are relatively poor when compared with natural hard tissue. Their poor mechanical properties, especially in aqueous environments, limit their applications to small, unloaded and lightly-loaded implants, powders, coatings, composites, and porous scaffolds for tissue engineering, and so on. One big advantage is that this material will degrade over time and will eventually be replaced by natural host calcium phosphates [18].

14.3 Biomaterial Constructs for Tissue Engineering: Scaffolds

The core of tissue-engineered grafts is hybrid constructs, which combine cells with biomaterial scaffolds. Cells and their products provide the primary biological functions, which are required and artificial materials provide the structural support and aids in mechanotransduction. The ideal results are a seamless integration of the grafts with the host, fully restored biological function and maintenance of smooth communication between the engineered tissue and the host. The artificial materials used for tissue engineering scaffolds can be polymers, ceramics, or composites and can be purely natural or fully synthetic. The trend in developing biomaterials for scaffolds includes the use of:

(1) temporary scaffolds, which gradually disappear after their intended use is completed;

(2) smart materials, which can respond to stimulation of the biological environment [31];

(3) scaffold chemistry patterning, using protein stamping [32, 33], microfliudic patterning [34], or photochemical modification [35] to incorporate specific bioactive domains on the scaffold surface to promote cell adhesion, migration, and tissue ingrowth and repair;

(4) pulsatile delivery of drugs or bioactive molecules on demand [36]; and

(5) anti-nonspecific adsorption surfaces, which can block undesirable protein and cell adhesion [21, 27].

The ultimate goal in scaffolding studies is to create the ideal scaffold, which would not only provide structural support, but also exchange physicochemical signals with the surrounding cells and the host environment.

14. 3. 1   Definition and Requirements for Scaffolds Used in Tissue Engineering

A scaffold is an artificial three-dimensional frame structure that serves as a mimic of extracellular matrix for cellular adhesion, migration, proliferation, and tissue regeneration in three dimensions. Its architecture and microstructure define the ultimate shape and structure of the regenerated tissue and organs.

An ideal scaffold for tissue engineering should possess the following characteristics [3, 7, 19 − 21]:

(1) it is highly biocompatible and does not elicit an immunological or clinically detectable foreign body reaction;

(2) it is three-dimensional and capable of regenerating tissue and organs in their normal physiological shape;

(3) it is highly porous with an interconnected pore network available for cell growth and nutrient and metabolic waste transport;

(4) it has a suitable surface chemistry allowing for cell attachment, migration, proliferation, and differentiation;

(5) it has controllable degradation and resorption rates that match the rate of tissue growth *in vitro*, *ex vivo*, and *in vivo* for biodegradable or resorbable materials;

(6) it possesses the appropriate mechanical properties which match those of the normal tissue and organs; and

(7) it has a bioactive surface to encourage faster regeneration of the tissue.

14. 3. 2   Principles of Scaffold Design

All tissue and organs in the body are three-dimensional structures. In order to repair and regenerate lost or damaged tissue and organs, three-dimensional scaffolds must be designed, fabricated, and utilized to regenerate the tissue similar in both anatomical structure and function to the original tissue or organ to be replaced or repaired. Therefore, certain principles of scaffold design must be established to ensure proper tissue regeneration.

14. 3. 2. 1   Tensegrity Concept

Ingber proposed an important principle in scaffold design based on the tensegrity concept [38, 39]. The tensegrity concept sounds new, but it is not a brand new concept because it has been used for centuries in the area of civil engineering. The core of this concept is that mechanical forces are evenly distributed on all regions of the entire scaffold. Therefore, stable structures that can bear forces uniformly, such as triangles, pentagons or hexagons, are preferred structures in a scaffold.

14.3.2.2 Nutrient and Metabolic Concept

Any living thing needs to consume nutrients and release waste products in order to survive. To keep tissue-engineered grafts alive, the diffusion of nutrients and metabolic products into and out of the three-dimensional scaffold is a key parameter to maintain. Highly porous and interconnected structures have been employed to facilitate the transport of materials through the scaffolds. However, these measures are not sufficient for the regeneration of large tissue and organs, such as the regeneration of liver [7]. Unfortunately, there is not a good answer for this problem yet.

14.3.2.3 Neovascularized Network Concept

The neovascularized network concept is an advancement of the nutrient and metabolic concept. In order to ultimately solve the nutrient and metabolic problems of engineered tissues, well-organized and uniformly distributed blood vessel networks are required. However, the technology to construct sufficient blood vessel networks outside the body has not been established yet. So far, one vital obstacle in the creation of tissue-engineered whole organs is the inability to provide proper vascularization to the newly created tissue or organ. This problem is especially serious in the development of a tissue-engineered liver.

The longest possible distance from a cell to blood vessels necessary to keep the cells alive in most healthy tissue is less than 1 mm. Therefore, when designing a tissue or organ, the time frame of blood vessel development must be well thought-out. With knowledge of neovascularization obtained from developmental biology and cancer studies well established, this problem may finally be solved. Currently, most scientists are trying to incorporate angio-genic factors into scaffold design in order to encourage the formation of blood vessel networks in the grafts [40, 41].

14.3.3 Scaffold Fabrication Technologies

A number of scaffold fabrication technologies have been developed or adopted from other disciplines for tissue engineering. There are three basic categories: three-dimensional polymeric scaffold fabrication, fiber and textile fabrication, and inorganic scaffold fabrication.

14.3.3.1   Three-Dimensional Polymeric Scaffold Fabrication

These techniques including the stack method, solvent casting, spin casting, particulate leaching, supercritical-fluid gassing process, emulsion freeze drying, phase separation, fiber bonding, membrane lamination, melt molding, fused deposition modeling, and three-dimensional printing, and so on have been proposed and utilized in fabricating three-dimensional scaffolds from polymeric materials.

The Stack Method

The stack method is a very simple way to create a three-dimensional frame structure using small disks with notches, which allows for the stacking of the disks with each other into three-dimensional architectures [42]. This method is similar to the children's building practice using toy bricks. The assembled structure fulfills the tensegrity concept very well and has good mechanical support in the early stages of application. However, the problem with this method is that it requires use of a large amount of polymer in order to form a stable three-dimensional object. The use of too much material with biodegradable polymers is not desirable because it may produce abundant acidic by-products, which may disturb the local environment and affect cell viability and function.

Solvent Casting

Solvent casting is based on the evaporative property of some solvents in order to form scaffolds by one of two routes. One approach is to dip a mold into the polymer solution and allow sufficient time to draw off the solvent, which leads to the formation of a layer of polymeric membrane. The other way is to place the polymer solution in a mold, and allow sufficient time for the solvent to vaporize, which leaves behind a layer of membrane adhering to the mold. This technique is very simple, easy, and inexpensive and there is no need for specialized equipment and no large effects on the degradation behavior. However, it uses highly toxic solvents which can denature proteins and other incorporated molecules. There is also the possibility for retention of toxic solvent within the scaffold, although this can be overcome by allowing the scaffold to fully dry and by using a vacuum process to further remove any solvent. However, this is a very time consuming and labor intensive fabrication process [43]. Some researchers have combined other techniques with solvent casting to obtain more features in the scaffold and avoid the disadvantages with solvent casting. For example, when combined with particle leaching techniques, scaffolds with $20\% - 50\%$ porosity can be obtained. However, this process only works for the construction of very thin scaffolds. Otherwise, it is very difficult to completely dissolve the soluble porogen particles from the core of the scaffolds. If the scaffolds are too thick, particles may remain in the scaffold. One method to overcome this problem may be to use the lamination principle to glue multiple thin porous sheets into a thick three-dimensional architecture. However, this is a very time consuming process [43]. By combining solvent casting with phase inversion or separation, asymmetric porous structures may be obtained. By combining the solvent casting process with micropatterning, patterns can be transferred to the surface of the scaffolds [3].

Spin Casting or Spin Coating

Spin casting or spin coating is based on the same principles as solvent casting. It can be classified as a sub-type of solvent casting. Briefly, the polymer to be deposited is dissolved in a solvent in order to make a polymer solution. The substrate, usually a glass cover slip or a silicon wafer, is held by vacuum on a chuck. The solution is then applied to the substrate, which is rotated at an adjustable high speed. The solution spreads over the surface under centrifugal forces, which also causes some of the solvent to evaporate. A thin film of polymer is formed on the substrate. By varying a number of fabrication parameters, such as rotation speed, acceleration, spinning time, solution viscosity, and solution density, films with different thicknesses can be fabricated. However, the thickness that can be obtained is very limited [37].

Particulate Leaching

Leaching is one popular approach used in tissue engineering to fabricate porous scaffolds. Pores or channels are created using porogens, such as salt (NaCl), wax, or even sugar. Briefly, the polymer is dissolved in a solvent and porogens with the desired shape and size are placed into the mold with a previously determined arrangement. The solution is poured into the mold, which is filled with the porogen. Then the solvent is evaporated and the polymer/porogen composite is formed. The final step is leaching of the porogens by using an appropriate solvent. For example, water is used as the solvent to dissolve salt and sugar. By controlling the amount of porogen added and the shape and size of the porogens, scaffolds with different microstructures can be fabricated. Depending on the types of porogen used, there are three types of leaching techniques: particle leaching, ball leaching, and fiber leaching [43 – 45].

Supercritical Fluid Gassing Process

This technique is adopted from other areas as it has been used for decades in both the packaging industry and in the pharmaceutical industry. This technique is based on the fact that polymers can be plasticized when employing high-pressure gas, such as nitrogen or carbon dioxide. The viscosity of the polymer will decrease when the gas diffuses into and becomes dissolved in the polymer. The biggest advantage of this technique is that polymers can be processed at normal body temperatures, which allows for the incorporation of heat-sensitive drugs and biological agents. Another advantage is that a high porosity, of up to 90% with pore sizes ranging from 50 − 400 μm, can be easily obtained [46]. However, only polymers with a high amorphous fraction can be processed using this technique and only about 10% −30% of the pores are interconnected, which may be overcome by combining this technique with particle leaching to gain a highly interconnected network [46].

Emulsion Freeze Drying

This technique is based on immiscibility, like with water and oil, among some solvents, which can be called solvent non-solvent pairs. In short, the polymer is dissolved into a solvent and then a non-solvent is added. The solution is then mixed well to form an emulsion mixture. This mixture is poured into a mold and quenched under low temperature or by using liquid nitrogen. The frozen mixture undergoes a freeze-drying process to remove both the solvent and non-solvent. The advantages of this process are that greater than 90% porosity with pore sizes ranging from 15 −200 μm can be obtained. The pores are highly interconnected which is good for nutrient supply, metabolic waste clearance, cellular ingrowth, and vascularization. However, this technique is user-, equipment-, and technique-sensitive and the processing parameters have to be well controlled [47].

Phase Separation or Phase Inversion

As opposed to the emulsion freeze-drying technique, phase separation is based on the miscibility of the solvent and non-solvent pair of the polymer. Briefly, the polymer is dissolved into a solvent, and then the polymer solution is delivered to a non-solvent bath and the polymer is precipitated to form membranes, microspheres, or porous scaffolds. This technique has been extensively applied to fabricate hollow fiber membranes and microspheres, which allows for the incorporation of pharmaceutical and biological agents and even cells and tissues into the membranes and microspheres. By varying several fabrication parameters, such as the solvent non-solvent pair, polymer concentration, temperature, small molecular additives, and flow rate, different micro- and macro-structures can be obtained. However, similar to the emulsion freeze-drying technique, the phase separation technique is user-, equipment- and technique-sensitive and the processing parameters must be well controlled [48]. Combining this technique with gelatin, solvent exchange, and freeze-drying techniques, highly porous (up to 98%), three dimensional, nano-size fibrous matrices can be produced [45]. Another interesting variation of this technique is using water-soluble filaments, such as sugar filaments, to fabricate three-dimensional scaffolds with a nano-scale fibril structure and interconnected macroporous channels, which may be useful for eliciting cell migration deep into the matrix and providing for better transport properties of the scaffold [49].

Rapid Prototyping or Solid Freeform Fabrication

Rapid prototyping (RP), also called solid freeform fabrication (SFF) and wafer stacking system (WSS), refers to a class of technologies that uses Computer-aided design (CAD) data to fabricate three-dimensional objects. This technology can be viewed as a three-dimensional printer. The prototype is created using a computer and the data can be transferred to the three-dimensional printer, which "prints" out the designed scaffold. This is especially advantageous when designing complicated objects [50]. The biggest advantage with RP is the dramatic savings in time and money needed to develop a complex new type of scaffold. Up to now, at least five different RP techniques are commercially available [50]:

(1) stereolithography — The computer-controlled laser beam is used to solidify liquid polymers and the objects are built up layer by layer;

(2) selective laser sintering — The computer-controlled laser beam is used to melt the powder materials and fuses the powder into solid objects, which are built up layer by layer;

(3) laminated object modeling — The computer controlled laser beam is used to cut out shapes layer by layer and the layers are glued together to form a three-dimensional structure;

(4) Fused deposition modeling (FDM) — Polymer is extruded from a nozzle and guided to the desired position *via* computer control. Each layer is then fused together before the polymer solidifies;

(5) Three-dimensional printing — A binder is "printed" out through a nozzle onto a powder bed to glue the desired amount of powder. The powder is then glued layer by layer until a three-dimensional object is formed. One advantage is that it allows for custom-made biological-synthetic hybrid scaffolds to be constructed because the entire process is performed at room temperature. Biological agents, such as cells and biomolecules, can be "printed" with binder to form a three-dimensional scaffold without sacrificing the cells and denaturing the biomolecules if a non-toxic binder, such as water, is used. The problem with this process is that it is difficult to find a non-toxic binder for most biomedical polymers [51].

14.3.3.2   Fiber and Textile Fabrication

The textile industry is very old and many technologies have been developed for processing woven or non-woven fabrics. Textile techniques have been adopted for the fabrication of tissue engineering scaffolds. For example, fibrous scaffolds have been created for engineering cartilage, tendons, bone, heart valves, blood vessels, nerves, and so on. Examples of fiber and textile fabrication techniques include fiber bonding and fused deposition modeling.

Fiber Bonding

One big advantage of using fibers is that they provide a very large usable surface area, which is desirable for scaffold applications because it provides more surfaces for cells to attach to. By simply piling the fibers together, three-dimensional scaffolds can be obtained. However, the scaffolds constructed using this method lack structural stability. To improve the stability, the fiber bonding technique may be used. This technique involves use of a binder, which has a non-common solvent to the fiber material, or, by using the thermal method to fuse the fibers together. A further development in this approach is to spray thick binder to form three-dimensional tubular scaffolds for the formation of blood vessels, intestines, and ureter tissue [31].

Rapid Prototyping Textiles: Fused Deposition Modeling

Rapid prototyping (RP) can be used not only with polymers, but with textiles as well, with the typical example being fused deposition modeling (FDM). Like other RP techniques, FDM forms three-dimensional objects from a digital file of CAD or any imaging source, such as computer-tomography (CT) and nuclear magnetic resonance imaging (NMRI). In brief, fibers are extruded from the head of a thermal extruder in a semi-liquid state, directed precisely to the desired position, and fused with other fibers during a solidification process. A computer-controlled platform with accurate X, Y, and Z movement, which determines the resolution of the equipment, is employed [52].

14.3.3.3   Inorganic Scaffold Fabrication

Porous bioceramics, such as hydroxyapatite (HA), tricalcium phosphate (TCP), and Bioglass®, have been developed for hard tissue implants and tissue engineering scaffolds, owing to their excellent material properties. These properties include excellent biocompatibility and bioactivity, bioresorption in calcified tissue, macroporosity, which facilitates cell and tissue ingrowth, as well as nutrient and waste product transport and vascularization [53]. There are basically two routes to fabricate three-dimensional biominerals scaffolds, which vary according to the temperature applied.

The High Temperature Route

The high temperature route is adopted from a traditional ceramic processing technique. This route for fabricating highly porous bioceramic scaffold consists of four steps. The first step is mixing the bioceramic raw powders with polymeric fillers. The polymeric fillers must be burned out completely in order to leave behind only non-toxic gases. The appropriate amount, size, and shape of the polymeric fillers determine the three-dimensional architecture, macrostructure, and microstructure of the scaffolds. The second step is compressing the mixture under pressure into the desired shape. The third step is burning of the polymer at a certain temperature for a particular time period. The final step is sintering the ceramic powder into a porous solid form. Through this high temperature route, scaffolds with a porosity of up to 70% can be obtained [54, 55]. However, the biggest problem with this method is that with increasing porosity, the mechanical properties of the scaffold decrease dramatically. By combining this method with hot isostatic processing (HIP) and nanotechnology, the mechanical properties of the porous ceramic scaffolds may be improved to some extent. Even with these modifications, porous bioceramics are generally still not strong enough for load-bearing situations, owing to their brittle nature.

The Low Temperature Route

Using the high temperature route, only macroporous ceramic scaffolds can be fabricated. However, Walsh developed a process called the bicontinuous microemulsion technique or crystal tectonics, which allows for the fabrication of porous scaffolds that are either mesoporous or macroporous. This technique is based upon the immiscibility phenomenon of emulsion similar to that used in emulsion freeze-drying techniques. Briefly, the scaffolds can be formed from oil-water-surfactant microemulsions supersaturated with biominerals. The pore size and structure are determined by the relative concentrations of water and oil [56, 57]. This proposed mechanism for the formation of highly porous complex structures is proposed in the following reference [56]. Since there is no report of the use of this material form as a scaffold for tissue engineering of any artificial organs, further investigation of biocompatibility issues and cell behavior on these surfaces needs to be done. Such complex, three-dimensional architectures with either mesoporous or macroporous structures may be utilized as scaffolds for tissue engineering organs, such as bone, as well as for other important applications such as lightweight ceramics, catalyst supports, biomedical implants, and robust membranes for high temperature separation technology.

In summary, all these techniques for scaffold fabrication are sensitive to the various processing parameters. For example, the choice of solvent in phase separation or inversion [48], controlled ice crystal formation and subsequent freeze-drying to create pores [58], and doping with porogen or leachants to generate pores [59] all affect both the microstructure and mechanical properties of the scaffolds.

14.4 References ˉ

1. Caplan, A. I. Tissue engineering designs for the future: new logics, old molecules. Tissue Eng. **6**(1): 1 −8(2000)

2. Ibarra, C., J. A. Koski, and R. F. Warren. Tissue engineering meniscus: cells and matrix. Orthop Clin North Am. **31**(3): 411 −418(2000)

3. Atala, A. Tissue engineering of artificial organs. J Endourol. **14**(1): 49 −57

4. Eaglstein, W. H. and V. Falanga. Tissue engineering and the development of Apligraf a human skin equivalent. Adv Wound Care. **11**(4 Suppl): 1 −8(1998)

5. Boyan, B. D., et al. Bone and cartilage tissue engineering. Clin Plast Surg, 1999. **26**(4): 629 −645(1999)

6. Ohshima, N., K. Yanagi, and H. Miyoshi. Development of a packed-bed type bioartificial liver: tissue engineering approach. Transplant Proc. **31**(5): 2016 −2017(1999)

7. Mayer, J., et al. Matrices for tissue engineering-scaffold structure for a bioartificial liver support system. J Controlled Release. **64**(1 −3): 81 −90(2000)

8. Mayer, J. E., Jr., T. Shin'oka and D. Shum-Tim. Tissue engineering of cardiovascular structures. Curr Opin Cardiol. **12**(6): 528 −532(1997)

9. Oberpenning, F., et al. De novo reconstitution of a functional mammalian urinary bladder by tissue engineering [see comments]. Nat Biotechnol. **17**(2): 149 −155(1999)

10. Tziampazis, E. and A. Sambanis. Tissue engineering of a bioartificial pancreas: modeling the cell environment and device function. Biotechnol Prog. **11**(2): 115 −126 (1995)

11. Mohammad, J., et al. Modulation of peripheral nerve regeneration: a tissue-engineering approach. The role of amnion tube nerve conduit across a 1-centimeter nerve gap. Plast Reconstr Surg. **105**(2): 660 −666(2000)

12. Germain, L., et al. Reconstructed human cornea produced in vitro by tissue engineering. Pathobiology. **67**(3): 140 −147(1999)

13. DiEdwardo, C. A., et al. Muscle tissue engineering. Clin Plast Surg. **26**(4): 647 − 656(1999)

14. Ratner, B. D. Biomaterials science : an introduction to materials in medicine. San Diego: Academic Press. 1 −63(1996)

15. Shinto, Y., et al. Calcium hydroxyapatite ceramic used as a delivery system for antibiotics. J Bone Joint Surg Br. **74**(4): 600 −604(1992)

16. Nolan, P. C., D. J. Wilson and R. A. Mollan. Calcium hydroxyapatite ceramic delivery system. J Bone Joint Surg Br. **75**(2): 334 −335(1993)

17. De Diego, M. A., N. J. Coleman and L. L. Hench, Tensile properties of bioactive fibers for tissue engineering applications. J Biomed Mater Res. **53**(3): 199 −203(2000)

18. Szivek, J. A. Bioceramic coatings for artificial joint fixation. Invest Radiol. **27**(7): 553 −558(1992)

14. 4 References

19. Peter, S. J. , et al. Polymer concepts in tissue engineering. J Biomed Mater Res. **43**(4): 422 –427(1998)

20. Cima, L. G. , et al. Tissue engineering by cell transplantation using degradable polymer substrates. J Biomech Eng. **113**(2): 143 –151(1991)

21. Hubbell, J. A. Biomaterials in tissue engineering. Biotechnology (N Y). **13**(6): 565 – 576(1995)

22. Ma, P. X. , et al. Engineering new bone tissue in vitro on highly porous poly(alpha-hydroxyl acids)/hydroxyapatite composite scaffolds. J Biomed Mater Res. **54**(2): 284 – 293(2001)

23. Silver, F. H. and G. Pins. Cell growth on collagen: a review of tissue engineering using scaffolds containing extracellular matrix. J Long Term Eff Med Implants. **2**(1): 67 –80(1992)

24. Kemp, P. D. Tissue engineering and cell-populated collagen matrices. Methods Mol Biol. **139**: 287 –293(2000)

25. Chang, R. K. and J. C. Price. Aliphatic polyesters and cellulose-based polymers for controlled release applications. J Biomater Appl. **3**(1): 80 –101(1988)

26. Li, S. Hydrolytic degradation characteristics of aliphatic polyesters derived from lactic and glycolic acids. J Biomed Mater Res. **48**(3): 342 –353(1999)

27. Vert, M. , et al. Bioresorbability and biocompatibility of aliphatic polyesters. J. Mater. Sci. **3**: 432 –446(1992)

28. Bruck, R. , et al. Non – peptidic analogs of the cell adhesion motif RGD prevent experimental liver injury. Isr Med Assoc J. **2** Suppl: 74 –80(2000)

29. Bruck, R. , et al. The use of synthetic analogues of Arg-Gly-Asp (RGD) and soluble receptor of tumor necrosis factor to prevent acute and chronic experimental liver injury. Yale J Biol Med. **70**(4): 391 –402(1997)

30. Ojima, I. , S. Chakravarty and Q. Dong. Antithrombotic agents: from RGD to peptide mimetics. Bioorg Med Chem. **3**(4): 337 –360(1995)

31. Gan, D. and L. A. Lyon. Tunable swelling kinetics in core — shell hydrogel nanoparticles. J Am Chem Soc. **123**(31): 7511 –7517(2001)

32. Patel, N. , et al. Printing patterns of biospecifically – adsorbed protein. J Biomater Sci Polym Ed. **11**(3): 319 –331(2000)

33. Okabe, Y. , et al. Chemical force microscopy of microcontact-printed self-assembled monolayers by pulsed – force – mode atomic force microscopy. Ultramicroscopy. **82**(1 – 4): 203 –212(2000)

34. Delamarche, E. , et al. Patterned delivery of immunoglobulins to surfaces using microfluidic networks. Science. **276**(5313): 779 –781(1997)

35. Park, Y. J. , et al. Controlled release of platelet-derived growth factor from porous poly (L-lactide) membranes for guided tissue regeneration. J Controlled Release. **51**(2 – 3): 201 –211(1998)

36. Benghuzzi, H. , R. Possley and B. England. Pulsatile delivery of progesterone and estradiol to mimic the ovulatory surge in adult ewes by means of TCPL implants. Biomed Sci Instrum. **30**: 187 –195(1994)

37. Lanza, R. P. , R. S. Langer and J. Vacanti. Principles of tissue engineering. 2nd ed. San Diego: Academic Press. 1 –73(2000)

38. Ingber, D. E. Tensegrity: the architectural basis of cellular mechanotransduction. Annu Rev Physiol. **59**: 575 –599(1997)

39. Chen, C. S., et al., Geometric control of cell life and death. Science. **276**(5317): 1425 – 1428(1997)

40. Elcin, Y. M., V. Dixit, and G. Gitnick. Extensive in vivo angiogenesis following controlled release of human vascular endothelial cell growth factor: implications for tissue engineering and wound healing. Artif Organs. **25**(7): 558 – 565(2001)

41. Lee, H., et al. Local delivery of basic fibroblast growth factor increases both angiogenesis and engraftment of hepatocytes in tissue-engineered polymer devices, Transplantation. **73**(10): 1589 – 1593(2002)

42. Hutmacher, D. W. Scaffolds in tissue engineering bone and cartilage. Biomaterials. **21**(24): 2529 – 2543(2000)

43. Mikos, A. G., et al. Laminated three – dimensional biodegradable foams for use in tissue engineering. Biomaterials. **14**(5): 323 – 330(1993)

44. Freed, L. E., et al. Neocartilage formation in vitro and in vivo using cells cultured on synthetic biodegradable polymers. J Biomed Mater Res. **27**(1): 11 – 23(1993)

45. Ma, P. X. and R. Zhang, Synthetic nano-scale fibrous extracellular matrix. J Biomed Mater Res. **46**(1): 60 – 72(1999)

46. Mooney, D. J., et al., Novel approach to fabricate porous sponges of poly(D, L-lactic-co-glycolic acid) without the use of organic solvents. Biomaterials. **17**(14): 1417 – 1422(1996)

47. Wang, K., et al. Ectopic bone formation via rhBMP-2 delivery from porous bioabsorbable polymer scaffolds. J Biomed Mater Res. **42**(4): 491 – 499(1998)

48. Nam, Y. S. and T. G. Park. Porous biodegradable polymeric scaffolds prepared by thermally induced phase separation. J Biomed Mater Res. **47**(1): 8 – 17(1999)

49. Zhang, R. and P. X. Ma. Synthetic nano-fibrillar extracellular matrices with predesigned macroporous architectures. J Biomed Mater Res. **52**(2): 430 – 438(2000)

50. Park, A., B. Wu, and L. G. Griffith. Integration of surface modification and 3D fabrication techniques to prepare patterned poly(L-lactide) substrates allowing regionally selective cell adhesion. J Biomater Sci Polym Ed. **9**(2): 89 – 110(1998)

51. Giordano, R. A., et al. Mechanical properties of dense polylactic acid structures fabricated by three dimensional printing. J Biomater Sci Polym Ed. **8**(1): 63 – 75(1996)

52. Gray, I. V. R. W., D. G. Baird and J. H. Bohn. Effects of processing condition on short TCLP fiber reinforced FDM parts. Rapid Prototyping J. **1**: 14 – 25(1998)

53. Petite, H., et al. Tissue-engineered bone regeneration. Nat Biotechnol. **18**(9): 959 – 963(2000)

54. Li, S. H., et al. Synthesis of macroporous hydroxyapatite scaffolds for bone tissue engineering. J Biomed Mater Res. **61**(1): 109 – 120(2002)

55. Nordstrom, E., et al. Osteogenic differentiation of cultured marrow stromal stem cells on surface of microporous hydroxyapatite based mica composite and macroporous synthetic hydroxyapatite. Biomed Mater Eng. **9**(1): 21 – 26(1999)

56. Walsh, D. and S. Mann. Fabrication of hollow porous shells of calcium carbonate from self-organizing media. Nature. **377**: 320 – 323(1995)

57. Walsh, D., J. D. Hopwood and S. Mann, Crystal tectonics: construction of recticulated calcium phosphate frameworks in bicontinuous reverse microemulsions. Science. **264**: 1576 – 1578(1994)

58. Yannas, I. V., et al. Wound tissue can utilize a polymeric template to synthesize a functional extension of skin. Science. **215**(4529): 174 – 176(1982)

59. Mooney, D. J., et al. Design and fabrication of biodegradable polymer devices to engineer tubular tissues. Cell Transplant. **3**(2): 203 −210(1994)

14.5 Problems

1. What are the differences between tissue engineering and traditional biomaterials?

2. What are the basic components of tissue engineering?

3. What are the fundamental approaches of tissue engineering?

4. How does tissue engineering differ from cloning and genetic engineering?

5. What are the requirements for a material used for tissue engineering?

6. Which category of the biodegradable polymer is preferred for tissue engineering? Why?

7. How does varying the ratio of PGA to PLA influences the time of degradation of the co-polymer PLGA (Answer with a graph) ?

8. List the various types of biomaterials on a broad level.

9. List the factors that influence the degradation behaviors of biodegradable polymers.

10. What is a scaffold for tissue engineering? What are the requirements for an ideal scaffold?

11. Bone is a natural composite material. Briefly discuss the levels of hierarchy (from nm to mm) of bone structure.

12. You are designing a long-term (up to a year) drug delivery device which degradable polymer is best for your purpose?

13. Why would an orthopedic surgeon like to use degradable materials for bone fracture fixation?

14. Using graphical representation, show what is meant by the term "polymer degradation".

15. What factors influence the biocompatibility of an implant?

16. What is the main composition of bioactive glasses?

17. Why polymeric materials are the most preferred for tissue engineering applications?

18. What are two degradation schemes for biodegradable polymers? Please discuss the effect of sample size on the degradation scheme.

19. Discuss the potential problems associated with acidic products of synthetic biodegradable polymers.

15 Cells and Biomolecules for Tissue Engineering

15.1 Cells for Tissue Engineering

Cells are the core component in building and maintaining tissue function in both real tissue and engineered tissue. Selection of the correct cells to use is an important starting point for engineering any tissue or organ. Several things must be considered when selecting which cells to use, such as the type, quantity, quality (free of pathogens, free of contamination), and source of the cells. From the origin point of view, cells used for tissue engineering may be obtained from autologous, allogeneic, or xenogeneic sources.

Autologous cells are directly harvested from the same individual that the cells are implanted into. Owing to the lack of risk of immune rejection, autologous cells are the most desirable source of cells. However, most of the time, very few cells are available for harvesting from a donor patient, and the cells may not be in good shape if obtained from diseased tissue or from elderly patients [1].

Allogeneic cells are harvested from the same species as the host, but are taken from a different individual. Owing to the risk of immune rejection, immunosuppressive drugs or immunoisolation techniques are necessary when allogeneic cells are used [1].

Xenogeneic cells are harvested from a different species than the host. As with allogeneic cells, immunosuppressive agents or immunoisolation techniques are necessary due to the risk of immune rejection [1]. However, even if these immunosuppressive techniques are used, xenogeneic cells elicit a stronger inflammatory reaction than allogeneic cells [2].

In terms of their lifetime, cells may be either primary cells or immortal cell lines. Primary cells are directly harvested from living tissue. Through mechanical mincing, enzymatic digesting (trypsin, collagenase, papain, dispase, etc.), and purification, a cell suspension with desirable concentration can be obtained for future expansion, seeding and other purposes. Primary cells have a limited lifetime and have two possible fates: One is crisis, which means cells finally die. The other is the spontaneous transformation to immortal cells as a result of random mutations. Immortal cell lines are homogenous populations of cells obtained through transformation procedures. Therefore, they are immortalized, and can proliferate in culture indefinitely. If a population of immortal cells is derived from a single cell, it is called clonal cell line. Currently, commercial laboratories offer a variety of well-characterized immortal cell lines.

In terms of their potential, cells may be either differentiated cells or stem or precursor cells.

Tissue engineering is still in its early stages. Unfortunately, typical studies in this field still simply seed all kinds of cells on various types of porous scaffolds. Before any significant progress can be made in the field of tissue engineering, several issues related to the cells must be well characterized. These issues include the following: understanding the underlying mechanisms of cell migration, proliferation, and apoptosis; understanding how to maintain stability of differentiation; understanding the precise signal transduction pathways between cells and their supporting matrix and between cells and growth factors; and understanding how to transfer this knowledge to cell-scaffold interactions [1, 3, 4].

In order to recover the functions of the lost or damaged organs, cells used for tissue engineering must possess the proper phenotype and reach the appropriate functional state. For example, cells for engineering skin must be able to produce keratin, cells for engineering liver must be able to detoxicate, and cells for engineering cartilage must be able to produce matrix [1, 4, 5]. However, cells may lose their normal behavior when they are removed from their original environment [6]. One big challenge of tissue engineering is to fully understand how to maintain cell phenotype and normal functions. Because of the possibility of behavioral changes of cells when grown in culture, the fate of cells, which are transplanted back into the body, must be well understood. Particularly, immature cells, such as stem cells, have been shown to be tumorgenic in our lab. Cell proliferation and apoptosis are two very important issues in engineering tissue as well, because they are key processes in controlling the cellularity of an engineered graft [1].

The functions of individual cells are very important, but cell-cell interactions inside the grafts are vital as well because each tissue and organ has more than one function. Cell-cell interactions are very important for establishing normal histological microstructure and for maintaining all the functions of the engineered tissue. For normal tissue, contact inhibition and the genetic code control the gross morphology of the organ. However, the gross morphology of the engineered tissue is controlled by the shape of the scaffold that is used. There is no data so far, as to whether contact inhibition and genetic information in cells may be useful in controlling the gross morphology of an engineered organ.

Understanding cell-extracellular matrix (cell-ECM) interactions, such as how cells adhere to matrix in normal tissue, is important for acquiring the knowledge needed to control cell-scaffold interactions. Using this knowledge of cell-ECM interactions, one can adhere cells to scaffolds with a pre-designed pattern and arrangement to engineer tissue with the required complex structure. Knowledge of cell-ECM interactions is not only important for managing cell adhesion, but is also vital for controlling cell migration, proliferation, mechanotransduction, organization, and function [1]. For example, focal adhesion and signal transduction through the integrin receptor-cytoskeleton complex are vital for the exchange of signals between a scaffold and its cells, which influence cell spreading and patterning on the scaffolds [7]. At the same time, understanding cell-growth factor interactions is equally important for controlling cell behavior during regeneration [1]. Therefore, understanding all the possible interactions of cells with the microenvironment is the key to successfully engineering functional tissue.

During normal tissue formation and wound healing, cells are subjected to all kinds of dynamic forces, such as gravity, shear stress, compression, tension, vibration, and pressure. Previous studies have demonstrated that exposure to dynamic forces causes cell behavior to change. For example, under the force of tension, the rate of neurite outgrowth increases [8]. Under vibrational force, the secretion of collagen by fibroblasts also increases [9]. Under compressive force, the secretion of chondroitin sulphate proteoglycan (CSPG) by chondrocytes rises [10 – 12]. However, the underlying mechanism of how dynamic forces affect cell behavior and function is still unclear.

While various cells have been used in tissue engineering applications, there has been a recent focus on the unique capabilities of stem cells. Stem cells and precursors bring new hope to regenerative medicine. The two main advantages of stem cells are the ability to self-renew, which means they can reproduce themselves, and the ability to potentially differentiate into all the possible cell types [13, 14].

Stem cells may be harvested from two different sources for use in tissue engineering. Embryonic stem (ES) cells may be harvested from embryos and can be derived from germ cells as well. ES cells may serve as a good source of cells for tissue engineering applications if problems such as immune rejection and the high possibility of tumor genicity can be solved [1].

Stem cells can be harvested from adult tissue as well, such as from muscle, cartilage, bone, the nervous system, liver, pancreas, and adipose tissue [1]. However, stem cells are very rare in adult tissue. For example, there is only about one mesenchymal stem cell (MSC) per 100, 000 nucleated cells [15]. The big challenge of using stem cells in tissue engineering is to establish sophisticated protocols for stem cell isolation and expansion [13, 14, 16]. Like stem cells, precursor cells can differentiate into more than one cell type, but these cells have undergone some degree of differentiation [17]. For example, glial-restricted precursors (GRP) can differentiate into type I and type II astrocytes and oligodendrocytes, but not neurons [18]. Precursor cells can be harvested from adult tissue as well [16]. Transplantation of stem cells alone or in conjunction with primary cells has shown better regeneration than with use of primary cells alone [13 – 15, 19]. However, the results derived from using stem cells are very inconsistent. Simply transplanting stem cells without a thorough understanding of stem cell biology is not the ultimate solution. To successfully use stem cells and precursor cells in tissue engineering, several basic questions have to be answered. For example, how can one achieve a pure stem cell population in large amounts? How can one coerce stem cells to differentiate into the desired phenotype in high percentages? And are stem and/or precursor cells present in all tissues?

15. 2   Growth Factor Delivery in Tissue Engineering

Growth factors are proteins or polypeptides that can bind to receptors on the cell surface and transmit signals into the cell, primarily resulting in the modulation of various cellular activities, such as proliferation, differentiation, migration, adhesion, and gene expression [20, 21].

There are several interesting characteristic properties of growth factors. Some growth factors are stimulating. For example, platelet derived growth factor (PDGF) and epidermal growth factor (EGF) promotes proliferation of numerous cell types[22 – 24]. Some are inhibiting. For instance, transforming growth factor beta (TGF-β) inhibits macrophage and lymphocyte proliferation [25]. Some are either stimulating or inhibiting, depending on the condition. For example, fibroblast growth factor (FGF) can promote proliferation of many cell types, but inhibits the proliferation of some stem cells [19, 26]. Some growth factors are versatile in their effects on a variety of cells. For example, insulin-like growth factor-I (IGF-I) can promote the proliferation of numerous cell types[27, 28]. Some growth factors are quite specific, such as nerve growth factor (NGF), which can only promote neural cell activities. Many cell types can produce the same growth factor (e.g. platelets, endothelial cells and placenta cells can secrete PDGF [22, 29].) and the same growth factor can act on many different cell types with the same or different effects (e.g. PDGF can promote the proliferation of smooth muscle cells, glial cells, and connective tissue cells [22, 29]), which is called pleitropism [21]. Different growth factors can have the same biological effect on the same cells, which is called redundancy [21]. For example, both PDGF and EGF can promote the proliferation of glial cells [22, 30]. Depending on the distance between their sites of synthesis and their sites of action, growth factors can be classified as:

(1) endocrine, when the target cells are located away from the site of synthesis and factors are transported through the cardiovascular system;

(2) paracrine, when the target cells are nearby and factors diffuse to local regions;

(3) autocrine, when the target cells are the same cells that synthesized the growth factor;

(4) juxtracrine, when target cells and synthesis cells are in direct contact with each other, which is especially important in systems where diffusion is limited. For example, juxtracrines are more determinative than paracrines and endocrines in the nervous system;

(5) intracrine, when the growth factors and their receptors are inside of the same cell [20, 21].

Like the synthesis of many proteins, the synthesis of growth factors is initiated by gene transcription to form messenger ribonucleic acid-RNA (mRNA) and translation to form protein. Because their mRNAs are unstable, growth factors are not routinely stored and most have very short half-lives. Most new growth factor synthesis requires new mRNA and protein synthesis [20]. Soon after the synthesis, growth factors usually exist in either an inactive or partially active state, require proteolytic activation, and some of them may need to bind to other molecules to function [22].

There are four basic components in tissue engineering, with growth factors as one of them. Growth factors are very important in maintaining the phenotype of the seeded cells, influencing the regeneration of functional tissue, and further enhancing the integration and function of regenerated grafts with the host tissue. For example, TGF-β, bone morphogenetic protein-2 (BMP-2), and osteogenic protein-1 (OP-1 or BMP-7) can induce osteoblast differentiation while discouraging the development of fibroblast, adipocyte, or chondroblast phenotypes in a tissue engineered bone device [25, 31]. Therefore, growth factor delivery is one key for engineering healthy and functional grafts. There are two methods to deliver growth factors for the engineering of tissues. One is by adding growth factors to the media during culture *in vitro*. The other is by releasing the factors from a scaffold or from the transplanted cells. Polymeric and ceramic scaffolds can serve as carriers for growth factors or growth factor-releasing cells. Growth factors can be either directly mixed into scaffolds during fabrication or after fabrication in the form of microparticles, nanoparticles, pellets, or sticks [20], or placed into container-like scaffolds such as microspheres and hollow fiber membranes. Container-like scaffolds are advantageous for the encapsulation of growth factor-secreting natural or genetically engineered cells for the sustained delivery of growth factors [32, 33]. Cell encapsulation techniques have been used as a means for continuous growth factor delivery, as long as the cells remain viable, for the treatment of neurodegenerative diseases such as Parkinson's disease. The semipermeable polymeric membranes serve as immunoisolation barriers and are used to protect the encapsulated cells from being attacked by host immune components [32, 33]. For growth factors that are mixed into the scaffolds during fabrication, the growth factors are released by a diffusion-controlled mechanism if the polymers degrade through a bulk degradation process, which occurs with polyesters and polyurethanes. When surface erosion polymers such as polyanhydrides and polyorthoesters are used, the growth factors can be released by an erosion mechanism or a combination of this mechanism with diffusion.

Growth factor delivery is not the same for all growth factors or all tissues. The growth factor type, dosage, release pattern (constant, pulsatile, and time-programmed), kinetics of release, and duration of the delivery are all highly dependent on the type of tissue to be engineered [20]. For example, hormones are normally released in a pulsatile pattern. In order to achieve physiological releasing patterns, a pulsatile release pattern would be very beneficial. Pulsatile delivery patterns have been studied for insulin delivery, contraception, and growth promotion [34, 35].

Two of the main challenges in growth factor delivery are the very short lifetime of most growth factors and the low diffusion rate of growth factors in most living tissue. For example, the concentration of growth factors delivered to brain parenchyma decreases exponentially with distance from the implantation site [36 – 38]. In order to prolong the lifetime of delivered growth factors, conjugation techniques have been explored. For example, dextran-conjugated nerve growth factor (NGF) and polyethylene glycol (PEG)-conjugated NGF have been shown to extend the life span of NGF in brain tissue [36 – 38].

15.3 Regulatory Matrix Proteins

Tissue is not solely composed of cells, as the extracellular matrix (ECM) is another important component that fills the space not occupied by cells. The ECM is a natural scaffold with a highly organized architecture, which surrounds and supports the cells in tissue. Their major role includes modulating cell behavior such as morphogenesis, migration, differentiation, and proliferation [39]. The ECM is composed of various proteoglycans, polysaccharides, and proteins and can be classified into three major categories: fibrous proteins (also called structural proteins; e.g. collagen and elastin), adhesion proteins (e.g. fibronectin (FN), and laminin (LN)), and glycosaminoglygans (GAG's, e.g. hyaluronan) and proteoglycans.

Collagens are the most abundant ECM molecules in the body and are primarily synthesized by fibroblasts and their family of cells, such as chondrocytes in cartilage, osteoblasts in bone, adipocytes in fat, and epithelial cells. Although over 20 types of collagen have been identified, they all possess the same core structure: three α-chain polypeptides that form coiled units, which wind around each other. One important function of collagen is that it affects cell differentiation. For example, when there is direct contact with the collagen produced by the lens in the eye, corneal epithelial cells continue to differentiate. Otherwise, corneal epithelial cells stop differentiating [40]. Hauschka demonstrated that interstitial collagen can promote myoblasts to differentiate into myotubes [41, 42].

The main function of elastin is to provide elasticity and resilience to tissue. Due to its high content of hydrophobic amino acids, such as valine, alanine, leucine, and glycine, elastin is one of the most chemically—and proteinase-resistant proteins in the body. The molecules are able to slide over one another and stretch or shrink extensively to provide elasticity and resilience. Elastin also promotes cell adhesion and can be chemotactic.

Depending on their location or form, there are two types of fibronectins (FN). One is plasma fibronectin, which circulates in body fluids to enhance blood clotting and phagocytosis. The other is insoluble fibronectin, which sticks on cell surfaces and deposits to interstitial spaces, such as the ECM. FNs are dimers with more than six tightly folded domains and can attach cells to surrounding matrix due to their possession of the cell surface-binding amino acid sequence arginine-glycine-aspartate (RGD). The main functions of the ECM form of FN are to modulate cell growth, differentiation, and migration during development [43, 44].

LN is composed of three chains and assembles into a cruciform molecule with one long arm and three short arms. Owing to their interchangeable chain structures, there are 18 different LN iso-forms. LN plays an important role in development, differentiation, and migration due to its interaction with cells through integrins on cell surfaces [43, 44].

GAG's are polysaccharides made up of repeating disaccharide units of amino sugar derivatives. Due to their highly hydrated nature, GAG's form gel-like structures in tissue. Fibrous proteins are embedded into and covalently bonded to the GAG's. Depending on the types of sugar residues and linkages between these residues, as well as the number and location of the sulphate groups, GAG's are classified into four types: chondroitin sulphate and dermatan sulphate, heparin sulphate and heparin, keratan sulphate, and hyaluronan.

Extracellular matrix(ECM) molecules are very important for normal cell behavior. Therefore, it is advantageous to incorporate ECM molecules in the development of functional tissue. Several factors must be considered in this design. For example, the proper substrate for normal cell behavior, including morphogenesis, migration, differentiation, and proliferation, is essential. ECM molecules or ECM analogues, which may affect cell behavior from the beginning of culture to the functional stage, are utilized in scaffold design and tissue culture. However, whole ECM molecules are immunogenic and may cause inflammation and even rejection. One solution is to identify short functional peptide sequences from the ECM, synthesize these short peptides, and then combine them with a non-immunogenic scaffold to function as an artificial ECM [45 −47].

15.4　References

1. Good, T. Current research in cell and tissue engineering. IEEE Eng. Med. Biol. Mag. **17**: 16, 18 (1998)
2. Rihova, B. Immunocompatibility and biocompatibility of cell delivery systems. Adv. Drug. Deliv. Rev. **42**: 65 −80 (2000)
3. Kehe, K., M. Abend, R. Ridi, R. U. Peter, D. van Beuningen. Tissue engineering with HaCaT cells and a fibroblast cell line. Arch. Dermatol. Res. **291**: 600 −605 (1999)
4. Bruder, S. P., B. S. Fox. Tissue engineering of bone. Cell based strategies. Clin. Orthop. S68 −83 (1999)
5. Wang, T. G. New technologies for bioartificial organs. Artif. Organs **22**: 68 − 74 (1998)
6. Ibarra, C., J. A. Koski, R. F. Warren. Tissue engineering meniscus: cells and matrix. Orthop Clin. North Am. **31**: 411 −418 (2000)
7. Ingber, D. E. Tensegrity: the architectural basis of cellular mechanotransduction. Annu. Rev. Physiol. **59**: 575 −599 (1997)
8. Smith, D. H., J. A. Wolf, D. F. Meaney. A new strategy to produce sustained growth of central nervous system axons: continuous mechanical tension. Tissue Eng. **7**: 131 − 139 (2001)
9. Webb, K., K. W. Broadhead, S. D. Gray, P. A. Tresco. Engineering the biomechanical properties of connective tissue matrix in porous, elastomeric biomaterials. In: 2003 Society For Biomaterials 29th Annual Meeting. p. 725 (2003)
10. Elder, S. H., S. A. Goldstein, J. H. Kimura, L. J. Soslowsky, D. M. Spengler. Chondrocyte differentiation is modulated by frequency and duration of cyclic compressive loading. Ann. Biomed. Eng. **29**: 476 −482 (2001)
11. Freeman, P. M., R. N. Natarajan, J. H. Kimura, T. P. Andriacchi. Chondrocyte cells respond mechanically to compressive loads. J. Orthop. Res. **12**: 311 −320 (1994)
12. Gray, M. L., A. M. Pizzanelli, R. C. Lee, A. J. Grodzinsky, D. A. Swann. Kinetics of the chondrocyte biosynthetic response to compressive load and release. Biochim.

Biophys. Acta. **991**: 415 – 425 (1989)

13. Pedersen, R. A. Embryonic stem cells for medicine. Sci. Am. **280**: 68 – 73 (1999)

14. Solter, D., J. Gearhart. Putting stem cells to work [see comments]. Science **283**: 1468 – 1470 (1999)

15. Bruder, S. P., N. Jaiswal, S. E. Haynesworth. Growth kinetics, self-renewal, and the osteogenic potential of purified human mesenchymal stem cells during extensive subcultivation and following cryopreservation. J. Cell Biochem **64**: 278 – 294 (1997)

16. Rizzoli, V., C. Carlo-Stella. Stem cell manipulation: why and how performing peripheral blood progenitor cell purging. Crit. Rev. Oncol. Hematol. **26**: 101 – 115 (1997)

17. Weissman, IL. Translating stem and progenitor cell biology to the clinic: barriers and opportunities. Science **287**: 1442 – 1446 (2000)

18. Foster, G. A., B. M. Stringer. Genetic regulatory elements introduced into neural stem and progenitor cell populations. Brain Pathol. **9**: 547 – 567 (1999)

19. Nevo, Z., D. Robinson, S. Horowitz, A. Hasharoni, A. Yayon. The manipulated mesenchymal stem cells in regenerated skeletal tissues. Cell Transplant **7**: 63 – 70 (1998)

20. Sheridan, M. H., L. D. Shea, M. C. Peters, D. J. Mooney. Bioabsorbable polymer scaffolds for tissue engineering capable of sustained growth factor delivery. J. Controlled Release **64**: 91 – 102 (2000)

21. Moorehead, B. *The Growth Factor*. College Press Pub. Co., Joplin, MO, p. 131 (1988)

22. Bowen-Pope, D. F., T. W. Malpass, D. M. Foster, R. Ross. Platelet-derived growth factor in vivo: levels, activity, and rate of clearance. Blood **64**: 458 – 469 (1984)

23. Eiselt, P., B. S. Kim, B. Chacko, B. Isenberg, M. C. Peters, K. G. Greene, W. D. Roland, A. B. Loebsack, K. J. Burg, C. Culberson, C. R. Halberstadt, W. D. Holder, D. J. Mooney. Development of technologies aiding large-tissue engineering. Biotechnol. Prog. **14**: 134 – 140 (1998)

24. Elcin, Y. M., V. Dixit, G. Gitnick. Extensive in vivo angiogenesis following controlled release of human vascular endothelial cell growth factor: implications for tissue engineering and wound healing. Artif. Organs **25**: 558 – 565 (2001)

25. Bonewald, L. F., S. L. Dallas. Role of active and latent transforming growth factor beta in bone formation. J. Cell Biochem. **55**: 350 – 357 (1994)

26. Lee, H., R. A. Cusick, F. Browne, T. Ho Kim, P. X. Ma, H. Utsunomiya, R. Langer, J. P. Vacanti. Local delivery of basic fibroblast growth factor increases both angiogenesis and engraftment of hepatocytes in tissue-engineered polymer devices. Transplantation **73**: 1589 – 1593 (2002)

27. Fansa, H., W. Schneider, G. Wolf, G. Keilhoff. Influence of insulin-like growth factor-1 (IGF-1) on nerve autografts and tissue-engineered nerve grafts. Muscle Nerve **26**: 87 – 93 (2002)

28. Elisseeff, J., W. McIntosh, K. Fu, B. T. Blunk, R. Langer. Controlled-release of IGF-1 and TGF-beta1 in a photopolymerizing hydrogel for cartilage tissue engineering. J. Orthop Res. **19**: 1098 – 1104 (2001)

29. Park, Y. J., Y. Ku, C. P. Chung, S. J. Lee. Controlled release of platelet-derived growth factor from porous poly(L-lactide) membranes for guided tissue regeneration. J. Controlled Release **51**: 201 – 211 (1998)

30. Drake, C. J., J. E. Hungerford, C. D. Little. Morphogenesis of the first blood vessels. Ann. N. Y. Acad. Sci. **857**: 155 – 179 (1998)

15.4 References

31. Wang, J. S. Basic fibroblast growth factor for stimulation of bone formation in osteoinductive or conductive implants. Acta. Orthop. Scand. Suppl. **269**: 1 – 33 (1996)

32. Tresco, P. A. Tissue engineering strategies for nervous system repair in process citation. Prog. Brain Res. **128**: 349 – 363 (2000)

33. Tresco, P. A., R. Biran, M. D. Noble. Cellular transplants as sources for therapeutic agents. Adv. Drug. Deliv. Rev. **42**: 3 – 27 (2000)

34. Hoerstrup, S. P., R. Sodian, J. S. Sperling, J. P. Vacanti, J. E. Mayer, Jr. New pulsatile bioreactor for in vitro formation of tissue engineered heart valves. Tissue Eng. **6**: 75 – 79 (2000)

35. Benghuzzi, H., R. Possley, B. England. Pulsatile delivery of progesterone and estradiol to mimic the ovulatory surge in adult ewes by means of TCPL implants. Biomed. Sci. Instrum **30**: 187 – 195 (1994)

36. Krewson, C. E., R. Dause, M. Mak, W. M. Saltzman. Stabilization of nerve growth factor in controlled release polymers and in tissue. J. Biomater. Sci. Polym. Ed. **8**: 103 – 117 (1996)

37. Belcheva, N., K. Woodrow-Mumford, M. J. Mahoney, W. M. Saltzman. Synthesis and biological activity of polyethylene glycol-mouse nerve growth factor conjugate. Bioconjug. Chem. **10**: 932 – 937 (1999)

38. Belcheva, N., S. P. Baldwin, W. M. Saltzman. Synthesis and characterization of polymer-(multi)-peptide conjugates for control of specific cell aggregation. J. Biomater. Sci. Polym. Ed. **9**: 207 – 226 (1998)

39. Lanza, R. P., R. S. Langer, J. Vacanti. *Principles of Tissue Engineering,* 2nd edition. Academic Press, San Diego, p. xli, 995 , [1] l. of plates (2000)

40. Meier, S., E. D. Hay. Control of corneal differentiation by extracellular materials. Collagen as a promoter and stabilizer of epithelial stroma production. Dev. Biol. **38**: 249 – 270 (1974)

41. Hauschka, S. D., I. R. Konigsberg. The influence of collagen on the development of muscle clones. Proc. Natl. Acad. Sci. U. S. A. **55**: 119 – 126 (1966)

42. White, N. K., S. D. Hauschka. Muscle development *in vitro*. A new conditioned medium effect on colony differentiation. Exp. Cell. Res. **67**: 479 – 482 (1971)

43. Chamoux, E., A. Narcy, J. G. Lehoux, N. Gallo-Payet. Fibronectin, laminin, and collagen IV as modulators of cell behavior during adrenal gland development in the human fetus. J. Clin. Endocrinol. Metab. **87**: 1819 – 1828 (2002)

44. Parmigiani, C. M., J. W. McAvoy. The roles of laminin and fibronectin in the development of the lens capsule. Curr. Eye Res. **10**: 501 – 511 (1991)

45. Bruck, R., R. Hershkoviz, O. Lider, H. Shirin, H. Aeed, Z. Halpern. Non-peptidic analogs of the cell adhesion motif RGD prevent experimental liver injury. Isr. Med. Assoc. J. **2** Suppl: 74 – 80 (2000)

46. Bruck, R., R. Hershkoviz, O. Lider, H. Shirin, H. Aeed, Z. Halpern. The use of synthetic analogues of Arg-Gly-Asp (RGD) and soluble receptor of tumor necrosis factor to prevent acute and chronic experimental liver injury. Yale J. Biol. Med. **70**: 391 – 402 (1997)

47. Ojima, I., S. Chakravarty, Q. Dong. Antithrombotic agents: from RGD to peptide mimetics. Bioorg. Med. Chem. **3**: 337 – 360 (1995)

15.5   Problems

1.   What is the amino acid sequence, "RGD"? Why is it significant?
2.   Name four types of bone replacements and briefly define them.
3.   Differentiate between the primary cells and immortal cell lines.
4.   Discuss the effects of dynamic forces on cell behaviors.
5.   Differentiate between the stem cells and precursor cells.
6.   What are the two different sources of stem cells?
7.   What is growth factor?
8.   What is pleitropism of growth factor? What is redundancy of growth factor?
9.   How to deliver growth factors for the engineering of tissues?
10. What is immunoisolation?
11. Please search the literatures, and discuss how to achieve a pulsatile pattern drug release?
12. What is ECM?
13. Why elastin is one of the most chemically- and proteinase-resistant proteins in the body?
14. How to deal with the modulation function and immunogenic possibilities of ECM molecules?

16 Transport and Vascularization in Tissue Engineering

16.1 Transport in Engineered Tissue

The transport of substances in all forms, such as solid, liquid, and gas, throughout tissue and organs is very important for maintaining normal living cells in engineered grafts. Transport in tissue engineering has two main issues: to design tissue with a well-perfused transport network and to create tissues, which would have the function of transport, such as cell encapsulation devices and blood vessels. There is no big difference between the concept of transport in tissue engineering and that found in classical chemical engineering. Like transport in the separation industry, molecular size and stereo-configurations determine the mechanism of transport. For example, in order to transport molecules from media into the cells, small molecules like oxygen and carbon dioxide can be transported through diffusion and convection mechanisms. Simple molecules, like some nutrients, are transported through diffusion and convection processes as well. Large molecules, like some growth factors and large proteins, have to be transported through receptor-mediated endocytosis [1,2]. In the biosystem, it is necessary to have bidirectional transport. For example, in order to keep the tissue and organs alive, oxygen, nutrients, and bigger biomolecules are transported into the tissue, and at the same time, metabolic products such as carbon dioxide and waste products are eliminated from the tissue. Therefore, perfusion of the engineered tissue is particularly important. To properly perfuse large organs, such as kidney and liver, diffusion and convection alone cannot meet the requirements. A well-established vascular network is essential. However, techniques to grow a blood vessel network throughout the tissue have not been developed. Therefore, semipermeable hollow fiber membranes (HFMs) have been employed to improve the transport properties of engineered tissue. For instance, HFM-based tissue-engineered kidney and liver have shown improved tissue perfusion and cell viability [3,4]. Despite this, a pre-engineered blood vessel network is still a requirement for engineered tissue [5,6]. Future efforts in this area may relate to fabrication of semipermeable hollow fiber membranes with optimized transport and angiogenesis-promoting properties.

16.2 Vascularization

One vital obstacle in tissue engineering is an inability to keep large engineered tissue and organs alive during both *in vitro* culture and future transplantation into the host. This is especially significant for large complex tissue, such as kidney and liver. Studies have confirmed that, without nutrients supplied through blood vessels, a piece of tissue with a volume beyond a few cubic millimeters, may undergo central necrosis [7, 8]. Broadhead [9] has demonstrated that engineered tissue is subject to central necrosis when nutrient transport occurs through diffusive transport rather than through the supply of blood vessels, using an *in vitro* semipermeable HFM culture system. Results from tumor research have also demonstrated that tumors cannot grow beyond a few millimeters in size unless they grow their own blood vessels [10].

16.2.1 New Blood Vessel Formation

During normal tissue formation and tissue remodeling in the body, new blood vessels can form by one of two routes: angiogenesis or vasculogenesis. In angiogenesis, new blood vessels are formed by sprouting off the pre-existing blood vessels [11]. Briefly, when there is a need for new blood vessel formation, such as after hypoxia, the concentration of angiogenic factors rises above normal, there is an increased sensitivity to angiogenic factors [12], pre-existing vessels may undergo vasodilation, or there may be a reduction of the contact inhibition among adjacent endothelial cells. Endothelial cells, pericytes, and vascular muscle cells then proliferate and form a tube-like structure [11]. For vasculogenesis, which normally takes place during embryogenesis in developing organs, new blood vessels are formed from migrating endothelial cells and their progenitors, angioblasts. Briefly, during development, angioblasts differentiate into endothelial cells and aggregate to form tube-like structures. Then pericytes and vascular smooth muscle cells migrate to the tubes and form structural blood vessels.

Angiogenic factors are specific molecules that can promote vascular formation via either vasculogenesis or angiogenesis [7, 13]. For example, both vascular endothelial growth factor (VEGF) and fibroblast growth factor (FGF) have been shown to directly affect endothelial cells and promote angiogenesis in both physiological and pathological conditions. Platelet derived growth factor (PDGF), transforming growth factor beta (TGF-β), and angiopoietin (Ang) do not directly influence endothelial cells, but they do induce angiogenesis *in vivo* [7, 13].

16.2.2 Vascularization in Tissue Engineering

With the growing knowledge in understanding the vascularization process and the properties of angiogenic growth factors, three strategies have been pursued for the vascularization of engineered tissues [8, 14]: incorporation of angiogenic growth factors while using microparticles and microbeads as release carriers, *via* seeding of angiogenic factor-secreting cells [15], seeding of endothelial cells or endothelial cell progenitors (EEPC) with functional cell types [16], and prevascularization of the scaffold prior to functional cell seeding [17]. Moreover, in tissue engineering, successful vascularization not only depends on the supply of endothelial cells or precursor cells and angiogenic growth factors, but also depends highly on the porosity of the scaffolds. Several investigators have demonstrated that pore size is very important in influencing the rate of vascularization [18, 19].

So far, *via* the techniques listed above, angiogenesis has been successfully accomplished in tissue-engineered skin. However, tissue-engineered skin is only a few thin layers of cells and for future tissue engineering applications, one must still attempt to create a vascular network for larger organs, such as kidney and liver.

16.3 References

1. Ratner, B. D. Biomaterials Science: An Introduction to Materials in Medicine. Academic Press, San Diego, p. xi, 484 (1996)
2. Lanza R. P., R. S. Langer, J. Vacanti. Principles of Tissue Engineering, 2nd edition. Academic Press, San Diego, p. xli, 995[1] l. of plates (2000)
3. Davis, J. M., J. A. Hanak. Hollow-fiber cell culture. Methods. Mol. Biol. **75**: 77 – 89 (1997)
4. Takeshita, K., H. Ishibashi, M. Suzuki, T. Yamamoto, T. Akaike, M. Kodama. High cell-density culture system of hepatocytes entrapped in a three-dimensional hollow fiber module with collagen gel. Artif. Organs **19**: 191 – 193 (1995)
5. Minuth, W. W., J. Aigner, B. Kubat, S. Kloth. Improved differentiation of renal tubular epithelium in vitro: potential for tissue engineering. Exp. Nephrol. **5**: 10 – 17 (1997)
6. Mayer, J. E. Jr., T. Shin'oka, D. Shum-Tim. Tissue engineering of cardiovascular structures. Curr. Opin. Cardiol. **12**: 528 – 532 (1997)

7. Veikkola, T., M. Karkkainen, L. Claesson-Welsh, K. Alitalo. Regulation of angiogenesis via vascular endothelial growth factor receptors. Cancer Res **60**: 203 – 212 (2000)
8. Langer, R. Angiogenesis — biomedical technology. Exs **61**: 23 – 25 (1992)
9. Broadhead, K. W., R. Biran, P. A. Tresco. Hollow fiber membrane diffusive permeability regulates encapsulated cell line biomass, proliferation, and small molecule release. Biomaterials **23**: 4689 – 4699 (2002)
10. Sutherland, R. M., B. Sordat, J. Bamat, H. Gabbert, B. Bourrat, W. Mueller-Klieser. Oxygenation and differentiation in multicellular spheroids of human colon carcinoma. Cancer Res **46**: 5320 – 5329 (1986)
11. Gallin, J. I., R. Snyderman. Inflammation: Basic Principles and Clinical Correlates. 3rd edition, Lippincott Williams & Wilkins, Philadelphia, p. xxiv, 1335 (1999)
12. Hanahan, D., J. Folkman. Patterns and emerging mechanisms of the angiogenic switch during tumorigenesis. Cell **86**: 353 – 364 (1996)
13. Nakagawa, K., Y. X. Chen, H. Ishibashi, Y. Yonemitsu, T. Murata, Y. Hata, Y. Nakashima, K. Sueishi. Angiogenesis and its regulation: roles of vascular endothelial cell growth factor. Semin. Thromb. Hemost **26**: 61 – 66 (2000)
14. Langer, R. Delivery systems for angiogenesis stimulators and inhibitors. Exs. **61**: 327 – 330 (1992)
15. Eiselt, P., B. S. Kim, B. Chacko, B. Isenberg, M. C. Peters, K. G. Greene, W. D. Roland, A. B. Loebsack, K. J. Burg, C. Culberson, C. R. Halberstadt, W. D. Holder, D. J. Mooney. Development of technologies aiding large-tissue engineering. Biotechnol. Prog. **14**: 134 – 140 (1998)
16. Park, H. J., J. J. Yoo, R. T. Kershen, R. Moreland, A. Atala. Reconstitution of human corporal smooth muscle and endothelial cells in vivo. J. Urol. **162**: 1106 – 1109 (1999)
17. Fontaine, M., B. Schloo, R. Jenkins, S. Uyama, L. Hansen, J. P. Vacanti. Human hepatocyte isolation and transplantation into an athymic rat, using prevascularized cell polymer constructs. J. Pediatr. Surg. **30**: 56 – 60 (1995)
18. Wake, M. C., C. W. Patrick, A. G. Jr., Mikos. Pore morphology effects on the fibrovascular tissue growth in porous polymer substrates. Cell Transplant **3**: 339 – 343 (1994)
19. Lado, M. D., D. R. Knighton, M. Cavallini, V. D. Fiegel, C. Murray, G. D. Phillips. Induction of neointima formation by platelet derived angiogenesis fraction in a small diameter, wide pore, PTFE graft. Int. J. Artif. Organs **15**: 727 – 736 (1992)

16.4 Problems

1. What are the transport mechanisms in tissue?
2. How new blood vessels form?
3. What strategies have been studied for the vascularization of engineered tissues?
4. RGD is a short functional peptide sequence allowing cell recognition, even selective adhesion. Now you are developing a synthetic cardiovascular graft

with an immobilized adhesion ligand, a short peptide sequence similar to RGD, for endothelial cells coating on the interior surface of the graft to avoid the problems of thrombus formation, when the graft is implanted into cardiovascular system, endothelial cells from the neighboring natural tissue can migrate into the graft by selective adhesion on your peptide. Therefore, the success of this approach relies in part on whether the peptide sequence you choose is recognized by only endothelial cell integrins.

(a) Please search the literature to find at least one short peptide sequence possible for your project (Please give references).

(b) Design a small experiment to test your hypothesis below:
   The success of this approach relies in part on whether the peptide sequence you choose is recognized by only endothelial cell integrins.

(c) If the peptide is recognized by many types of integrins, what may happen in the graft?

(d) How may immobilization via physical adsorption alone affect your outcome? How may you improve the graft performance by enhancing immobilization techniques?

17 Host Response to Tissue Engineered Grafts

The host response to a tissue-engineered graft comes in two parts: the foreign body response to biomaterial scaffolds and the immune response to the biological components, namely cells, tissue, and biomolecules.

17.1 The Foreign Body Response to Synthetic Components

From the foreign body response point of view, there is no difference between biomaterials used for traditional medical applications and biomaterials used for tissue engineering, since in both cases, the materials must be compatible. Biocompatibility requires that materials are not toxic, elicit a minimal foreign body reaction, and are not carcinogenic, immunogenic, antileukotactic, or mutagenic. However, there are no synthetic materials which are absolutely biocompatible [1, 2]. Moreover, many factors such as implant size, shape, material composition, surface wettability, roughness, and charge influence the host response to implant [1, 3, 4].

Inside the body, there is an aqueous and corrosive environment which is often detrimental to most implanted materials. For example, after implanting a material for a certain amount of time, the biological environment may decrease its mechanical properties, change its dimensions due to swelling, undesirably degrade it by hydrolysis, enzymatic, microcrack, or crazing corrosion with metallic materials, leaching, calcification, wear, fatigue, or undesirable fouling [1, 2].

All materials possess properties that the host tissue does not accept "silently", such as morphological, chemical, mechanical, biological, and electrical characteristics that may elicit tissue and cellular responses composed of three main sequences: inflammation, wound healing, and the foreign body response. Shortly after implantation, capillaries close to the injury vasodilate and there is an increase in the permeability of endothelial cells, which causes swelling. A variety of cells migrate towards the site of injury, such as neutrophils which appear first and are mainly responsible for phagocytosis, and macrophages at early time points, and foreign body giant cells and fibroblasts at later time points. At the same time, inflammatory cells secrete various factors that mediate the inflammatory response and tissue remodeling process[1, 2]. In fact, both the short-and long-term responses to any implanted material, from the acute, sub-acute, and chronic inflammatory response to the foreign body reaction to fibrous encapsulation to hypersensitivity to rejection, are governed by the cell-mediated and humoral immune responses[1]. The difference between injury alone and implantation is the long-term foreign body reaction, which may persist at the tissue-implant interface for the lifetime of the implant. The main characteristics of the foreign body reaction are the presence of macrophages and foreign body giant cells and formation of fibrous encapsulation tissue [1, 2]. The only way to eliminate the foreign body reaction is to get rid of the implanted foreign material. Therefore, the use of biodegradable materials may provide an advantage to avoid a long-term foreign body reaction. However, there is no information so far about any disappearance of the foreign body response after implanted materials are completely degraded.

Implantation of foreign materials into the cardiovascular system leads to a more complicated inflammatory response than that listed previously. As soon as grafts are implanted in the cardiovascular system, plasma proteins such as albumin, fibrin, and globulins adsorb onto the implant surface and cause platelets and leukocytes to adhere to the surface, leading to the polymerization of fibrin and the formation of thrombin [1, 2]. Many techniques have been utilized to inhibit protein adsorption, fibrin formation, and clot formation such as polyethylene oxide (PEO)-polypropylene oxide (PPO)-PEO coatings [5], heparin coatings, and endothelial cell seeding on the implant surface [6 - 8]. Injury to endothelial cells on the inner surface of blood vessels may cause clotting as well. Therefore, gentle implantation of tissue engineering grafts into the cardiovascular system is very important to avoid damage to the endothelial cells.

17.2　Response to Biological Components

The biological components of a tissue-engineered graft may be composed of cells and molecules derived from the same host individual, from a different individual, or even from a different species. The most preferred source is cells and biomolecules taken from the same host individual because there is no immune response following transplantation. Sometimes there are not enough supplies from the patients themselves and thus, it is necessary to use biological components from another individual or from other species, which will elicit an immune response and cause rejection of the transplanted grafts. Just like the response to synthetic materials, both the cell-mediated and humoral immune response may be involved. Alloantibodies, xenoantibodies, complement components, and cytokines are the major immunotoxic substances involved in the immune response [9 – 11]. In order to avoid immune rejection and its subsequent killing of the transplanted cells, several approaches have been studied. One solution is to identify short functional sequences from the biomolecules of interest and then to synthesize short non-immunogenic sequences of the biomolecules to function as essential biomolecules [12 – 14]. To protect the transplanted cells, two other possible strategies have been proposed: cell encapsulation and creation of "universal donor cell lines" using cellular engineering and genetic engineering techniques.

Cell encapsulation is based on the use of size-selective polymeric membranes, which allow for the transport of molecules smaller than the molecular weight cut-off (MWCO) of the membranes, but restrict the passage of molecules larger than the MWCO. Because most antibodies and complement components are over 20 nm in size, membranes with pore sizes of less than 20 nm are desired for protection of the encapsulated foreign cells [15]. However, there are several problems pertinent to this strategy. One is the low short-term viability of encapsulated cells caused by acute and sub-acute inflammatory factors. To overcome this problem, a novel concept called space creation has been developed. Low long-term viability of encapsulated cells caused by a progressively increasing fibrous capsule formation due to the foreign body reaction and the decreasing transport of nutrients may also kill the encapsulated cells in the long run [2]. To overcome this problem, a membrane which promotes vascularization into the membrane wall is desired. Angiogenic factors and a porous surface architecture may be used. Zhang has demonstrated that pore size is a very important factor influencing the rate of vascularization at the membrane-tissue interface [16].

Another problem is the so called "antigen shedding" effect, caused by the leakage of encapsulated cell products or dead cell fragments, which may lead to the production of antibodies to kill the encapsulated cells [2].

Creation of universal donor cell lines may be the ultimate solution to protect the transplanted cells. Two possible ways to engineer the transplanted cells are to alter major histocompatibility complex genes and to develop a cell line genetically identical to the host cells by somatic cell or nuclear transfer [17, 18].

17.3 References

1. Ratner, B. D. Biomaterials Science: An Introduction to Materials in Medicine. Academic Press, San Diego, p. xi, 484 (1996)
2. Hubbell, J. A. Biomaterials in tissue engineering. Biotechnology (N. Y). **13**: 565 – 576 (1995)
3. Ibarra, C., J. A. Koski, R. F. Warren. Tissue Engineering Meniscus: Cells and Matrix. Orthop Clin. North Am. **31**: 411 – 418 (2000)
4. Boyan, B. D., C. H. Lohmann, J. Romero, Z. Schwartz. Bone and cartilage tissue engineering. Clin. Plast. Surg. **26**: 629 – 645, ix (1999)
5. Amiji, M., K. Park. Prevention of protein adsorption and platelet adhesion on surfaces by PEO/PPO/PEO triblock copolymers. Biomaterials **13**: 682 – 692 (1992)
6. Usui, A., M. Hiroura, M. Kawamura. Heparin coating extends the durability of oxygenators used for cardiopulmonary support. Artif. Organs **23**: 840 – 844 (1999)
7. van der Giessen, W. J., H. M. van Beusekom, M. H. Eijgelshoven, M. A. Morel, P. W. Serruys. Heparin-coating of coronary stents. Semin. Interv. Cardiol. **3**: 173 – 176 (1998)
8. Wang, Z. G., H. Zhang. Seeding of autogenous endothelial cells to inner surface of small-caliber dacron vascular prostheses. An experimental study on canines. Chin. Med. J. (Engl.) **102**: 606 – 613 (1989)
9. Colton, C. K., E. S. Avgoustiniatos. Bioengineering in development of the hybrid artificial pancreas. J. Biomech. Eng **113**: 152 – 170 (1991)
10. Rihova, B. Immunocompatibility and biocompatibility of cell delivery systems. Adv. Drug. Deliv. Rev. **42**: 65 – 80 (2000)
11. Wang, T. G. New technologies for bioartificial organs. Artif. Organs **22**: 68 – 74 (1998)
12. Bruck, R., R. Hershkoviz, O. Lider, H. Shirin, H. Aeed, Z. Halpern. Non-peptidic analogs of the cell adhesion motif RGD prevent experimental liver injury. Isr. Med. Assoc. J. **2** Suppl: 74 – 80 (2000)
13. Bruck, R., R. Hershkoviz, O. Lider, H. Shirin, H. Aeed, Z. Halpern. The use of synthetic analogues of Arg-Gly-Asp (RGD) and soluble receptor of tumor necrosis factor to prevent acute and chronic experimental liver injury. Yale J. Biol. Med. **70**: 391 – 402 (1997)
14. Ojima, I., S. Chakravarty, Q. Dong. Antithrombotic agents: from RGD to peptide mimetics. Bioorg. Med. Chem **3**: 337 – 360 (1995)
15. Uludag, H., P. De Vos, P. A. Tresco. Technology of mammalian cell encapsulation. Adv. Drug Deliv. Rev. **42**: 29 – 64 (2000)
16. Zhang, N. The adult brain tissue response to hollow fiber membranes of varying surface architecture with or without co-transplanted cells. Department of Bioengineering, Salt Lake City: University of Utah, pp. 140 (2003)
17. Pedersen, R. A. Embryonic stem cells for medicine. Sci. Am **280**: 68 – 73 (1999)

18. Solter, D., J. Gearhart. Putting stem cells to work. Science **283**: 1468 – 1470 (1999)

17. 4   Problems

1. What are the general responses of the host to a tissue-engineered graft?
2. Explain the term biocompatibility in your own words.
3. Describe the wound healing response after the implantation of a tissue-engineered graft.
4. Differentiate the wound healing response between bone implants and cardiovascular stents after the implantation into the host.
5. Immobilizing the synthetic polymer poly(ethylene oxide), PEO, on surfaces has been a successful means of reducing non-specific protein adsorption. Using the concept of osmotic pressure and activity of water, explain the mechanism by which PEO "repels" proteins.
6. Search the literature and give a brief summary about using surface coatings to reduce protein adsorption on an implant surface (please give at least two methods). Be sure to consider the role of the surface density of the coating, as well as give some thought to the conformation or phase behavior of the coating. For example, PEO chains are polymers which adopt random coil conformations in solution, but when closely packed on surface, they are no longer described as random coils.
7. Your co-worker has created a new protein repellant product to be used in cardiovascular applications. He tests the product by studying the adsorption of fibrinogen, a major coagulation protein, to a silicone surface coated with his product. To further mimic the *in vivo* scenario, he studies the adsorption of fibrinogen from the whole plasma by fluorescently labeling only fibrinogen. The fibrinogen adsorption kinetic curve is given below:

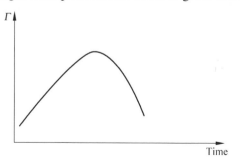

Upon seeing the decrease in adsorbed amount of fibrinogen after the initial increase, he exclaims, "It works — the surface repels fibrinogen, but only after a threshold level of fibrinogen is first adsorbed. " Knowing better, you tell him that similar behavior would likely to occur if he runs a control on untreated silicone.

(a) What, if not the surface coating, is leading to the fibrinogen desorption?

(b) Illustrate on the above graph what might be occurring.

8. Differentiate the host response to synthetic materials and biological components in the tissue-engineered grafts.

18 Other Important Issues and Future Challenges in Tissue Engineering

18.1 Organ Replacement and Regeneration

In order to replace the function of damaged or missing tissue and organs, two basic therapeutic strategies may be chosen. One is the transplantation of a replacement body part from the same individual, a living relative, a human cadaver, or a donor animal. The other is substitution of the tissue or organ with a man-made object, an implant, or artificial organ. Because there are many limitations associated with transplantation such as donor site morbidity and the immune response, the artificial organ approach becomes one promising route for treatment of organ failure.

There are two common methods used in the artificial organ approach. One method is replacement and the other is regeneration. In the replacement method, a biomaterial-based device is utilized solely to substitute the function of the damaged tissue, but there is no normal histological architecture recovery. For instance, metallic total hip prostheses are employed only to replace the load-bearing function of bone. In most replacement approaches, foreign materials are implanted into the body permanently. No matter how biocompatible the material is there will be an inflammatory response, foreign body response, and other problems associated with the material itself. In the regeneration method, tissue is guided to regenerate with the use of cells, scaffolds, growth factors, other bioactive factors, and dynamic forces. For example, growing tissue engineered cartilage using cells, scaffolds, and growth factors under force conditions leads to the formation of a functional and histological bone graft [1]. In regeneration techniques, the regenerative capacities of host cells or transplanted cells are awoken. Regenerated tissue and organs can avoid the problems associated with long-term foreign material implantation. Obviously, the regeneration approach is the ultimate choice of restorative medicine. In the future, regenerated tissue and organs may eliminate the replacement approach completely.

18.2　Organotypic and Histiotypic Models

Two-dimensional cell cultures are not desirable for engineering tissue and organs because both the histological organization and some physiological functions may be lost [2]. For example, there are many types of epithelia cells, such as keratinocytes, hepatocytes, kidney epithelial cells, and lung epithelial cells. When culturing any type of epithelial cell in a two-dimensional system, the cells lose their phenotype and cannot perform their normal functions. In order to overcome this, two models were developed: the organotypic model and the histiotypic model.

When culturing an entire organ or part of an organ such as thick slices of an organ, the organization and function of the organ can be retained. This is the so-called organotypic model [2]. This model can be used to study the development of many diseases. For example, thick slices of spinal cord or brain tissue have been used to study neurodegenerative diseases [3]. The advantages of this model may include the preservation of intact connections between neurons and they're supporting glial cells and maintenance of an environment for neurons which is comparable to normal. Generally, organotypic models may be used for a variety of applications including genomics, proteomics, drug delivery, and drug discovery research. The results obtained using this model may be very similar to those seen in a clinical trial, which is not possible with monolayer cell culture or traditional animal experiments. This model is an alternative to traditional animal testing. The problems with organotypic models include difficulties in the perfusion of whole explants, occlusion of blood vessels, necrosis of tissue in the center, a relatively short life span of the organ, and variable results caused by the previously listed factors [2].

The other model is an *in vitro* construct of tissue-like structures, which is made using cells, scaffolds, and biomolecules, and may include dynamic forces as well. This is called the histiotypic model. Many specific models have been established to mimic the function of real tissue, such as a skin equivalent model made using collagen gel, a vascular model made using collagen gel, and a bone tissue model made using collagen foam [2]. The advantage is that standard models can be easily established and these models may be used to overcome the variability problems seen with organ culture. However, the microstructure and function of these models are far from that of real tissue and organs [2].

Both models are useful in preliminary tests for drugs and toxins without having to use a large number of animals.

18. 3   Mechanotransduction

During normal tissue formation, tissue remodeling, and tissue functioning, cells and tissue not only generate forces, but are also subject to many kinds of physical forces such as gravity, shear stress, compression, tension, vibration, and pressure. Many but not all cell types and tissue can generate forces. For example, all kinds of muscle cells (myofibroblasts) can generate forces in many organs, such as skeletal muscle, smooth muscle in the gastrointestinal (GI) tract and blood vessels, and cardiac muscle in the heart. Surprisingly, all living cell types can sense forces and respond to these forces. Furthermore, there are some specific cell types called mechanosensory cells, whose main functions are to sense the forces. For example, sensory hair cells in the vestibular organs can sense shear force; alveolar endothelial cells and epithelial cells in the lungs can sense pressure and shear force; and osteoblasts and osteoclasts can sense mechanical stimuli to fine-tune bone remodeling.

However, cells cannot respond to any mechanical signal directly. In order for a cell to respond, mechanical signals must be converted into chemical signals. This conversion process is called mechanotransduction[4]. How cells convert mechanical signals into chemical responses is still unclear. Ingber has demonstrated that cells sense force through changes in the balance of the ECM-integrin-cytoskeleton complex, which is named the force transducing apparatus (FTA). When the balance of the FTA is changed, the secondary messenger system is initiated and this leads to synthesis of the appropriate protein. For example, when bone tissue is subjected to force, the balance of the FTA is distorted and the levels of cyclic adenosine monophosphate (cAMP), intracellular calcium, and prostaglandin E2 (PGE2) are increased. The rapid formation of stress fibers and focal adhesion complexes are initiated by an elevation in tyrosine phosphorylation and synthesis of actin-associated proteins [5]. Ingber has also demonstrated that all cell types adopt a tensegrity architecture for their organization, which indicates that all cell types have the capability to sense mechanical forces and self-adjust their own morphology, orientation, and even the arrangement of surrounding ECM molecules [4]. This information is particularly important for tissue engineering. To generate fully functional tissue and organs, a close mimicking of the normal growth conditions is desirable. However, when using a traditional static culture system, this is impossible to achieve. A dynamic culture system that supplies variable physiological stresses must be used. Unfortunately, the mechanical conditions or force environment needed and the mechanotransduction mechanisms during tissue formation and wound healing are not well understood. There are numerous questions left to be answered. For instance, how do forces affect morphogenesis during development? How do cells remodel organization of the ECM? How can myofibroblasts pull together the wound edge and close the wound? And what are the physiological force levels for different cell types at different developmental stages? To answer these questions, a dynamic culture system capable of production of all kinds, levels, and combinations of physiological forces has to be developed to study tissue formation, regeneration, and remodeling.

18.4 Future Challenges

Scientists have attempted to regenerate all kinds of tissues and organs including: blood vessels and other cardiac prostheses, corneas, pancreas, parathyroid glands, adrenal glands, the alimentary tract, liver, red blood cells, lymphoid cells, kidneys, bladders, the genitourinary system, bone, cartilage, tendons, ligaments, the auditory system, the visual system, nerves, spinal cord, brain, periodontal tissue, dentin, skin, and even an artificial womb. However, most research in tissue engineering is far from mature and is still in the early stages. Many challenges remain, including:

(1) creation of the ideal scaffold, which would not only provide structural support, but also exchange physicochemical signals with cells and the host environment;

(2) achieving a pure stem cell population in large numbers and obtaining a high percentage differentiation of stem cells to the desired phenotype;

(3) prolonging the lifetime of growth factors;

(4) avoiding immunogenic problems when using bioactive molecules and cells;

(5) achieving a desirable vascular network for larger organs, such as kidney and liver;

(6) creation of universal donor cell lines, which would not be rejected by the host;

(7) development of appropriate dynamic bioreactors to mimic the stress environment in normal tissue; and

(8) Studying the unknown fate of tissue-engineered analogues inside the human body.

Although many challenges lie ahead, tissue engineering, which is a very new area, is still very promising. The field of tissue engineering is to bring forth a new era of regenerative medicine.

18.5   References

1. Galletti, P. M. Organ replacement and regeneration. Cell Transplant **3**: S3 –4 (1994)
2. Lanza, R. P., R. S. Langer, J. Vacanti. Principles of Tissue Engineering, 2nd edition. Academic Press, San Diego, p. xli, 995 [1] l. of plates (2000)
3. Wang, M. Y., J. J. Kendig. Patch clamp studies of motor neurons in spinal cord slices: a tool for high — resolution analysis of drug actions. Acta. Pharmacol. Sin. **21**: 507 –515 (2000)
4. Ingber, D. E. Tensegrity: the architectural basis of cellular mechanotransduction. Annu. Rev. Physiol. **59**: 575 –599 (1997)
5. Hubbell, J. A. Biomaterials in tissue engineering. Biotechnology (N. Y.) **13**: 565 –576 (1995)

18.6   Problems

1. Differentiate between the terms "organ replacement" and "regeneration".
2. What are the limitations associated with tissue and organ transplantation?
3. Why 3D cell culture is needed to regenerate functional tissue-engineered grafts?
4. Differentiate between the terms " organotypic model" and " histiotypic model".
5. What is mechanotransduction?
6. What is FTA?
7. Read as many literatures in TE as possible, and try to bring out more challenges in TE research in the near future.

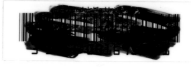